Introduction to
Research Methodology
for
Specialists and Trainees

Introduction to Research Methodology

for

Specialists and Trainees

Edited by
P M Shaughn O'Brien and
Fiona Broughton Pipkin

RCOG Press

First published 1999

© Royal College of Obstetricians and Gynaecologists 1999

ISBN 1-900364-11-5

Published by the RCOG Press at the
Royal College of Obstetricians and Gynaecologists
27 Sussex Place, Regent's Park
London NW1 4RG

Registered Charity No. 213280

RCOG editor: Jane Moody
Designed by Geoffrey Wadsley

Printed by Latimer Trend & Company, Plymouth

Contents

Contributors

Dr Sarah Ayres
Researcher, National Perinatal
Epidemiology Unit,
Radcliffe Infirmary,
Woodstock Road,
Oxford OX2 6HE

Professor Philip N. Baker
Professor of Obstetrics and
Gynaecology,
University of Nottingham,
Faculty of Medicine and Health
Sciences,
City Hospital, Hucknall Road,
Nottingham NG5 1PB

Dr Peter Brocklehurst
Unit Epidemiologist, National
Perinatal Epidemiology Unit,
Radcliffe Infirmary,
Woodstock Road,
Oxford OX2 6HE

**Professor Fiona Broughton
Pipkin**
Professor of Perinatal Physiology,
University of Nottingham,
Faculty of Medicine and Health
Sciences,
University Hospital, Nottingham
NG7 2UH

Dr Robin Burr
Specialist Registrar, Reproductive
Molecular Research Group,
Department of Obstetrics and
Gynaecology,
Queen Elizabeth Hospital,
Sheriff Hill, Gateshead,
Tyne and Wear NE9 6SX

Professor Linda Cardozo
Professor of Urogynaecology,
King's College Hospital,
Denmark Hill,
London SE5 9RS

Dr D. Stephen Charnock Jones
Lecturer, University of Cambridge,
Department of Obstetrics and
Gynaecology,
The Rosie Hospital, Robinson Way,
Cambridge CB2 2SW

Dr Paul W. Dimmock
Researcher, Academic Department
of Obstetrics and Gynaecology,
North Staffordshire Hospital,
Maternity Unit,
City General Hospital,
Newcastle Road, Stoke-on-Trent
ST4 6QG

Miss Lelia M.M. Duley
Obstetric Epidemiologist,
Magpie Trial Co-ordinating Centre,
Institute of Health Sciences,
Old Road, Headington,
Oxford OX3 7LF

Professor Cindy M. Farquhar
Associate Professor, Department of
Obstetrics and Gynaecology,
University of Auckland,
National Women's Hospital,
Claude Road, Epsom, Auckland,
New Zealand

Professor Nicholas M. Fisk
Institute of Obstetrics and
Gynaecology, Imperial College
School of Medicine,
Queen Charlotte's and Chelsea
Hospital, Goldhawk Road,
London W6 0XG

Dr Simon Gates
Trials Researcher/Statistician,
National Perinatal Epidemiology
Unit, Radcliffe Infirmary,
Woodstock Road,
Oxford OX2 6HE

Dr John M. Grant
Editor in Chief, British Journal of
Obstetrics and Gynaecology,
27 Sussex Place, Regent's Park,
London NW1 4RG

Dr Trish Greenhalgh
Senior Lecturer in Primary Health
Care, Unit for Evidence-Based
Practice and Policy,
Joint Department of Primary Care
and Population Studies,
Royal Free and University College
London Medical Schools,
Whittington Hospital, Highgate Hill,
London N19 5NF

Professor David A. Grimes
Clinical Professor, Department of
Obstetrics and Gynaecology,
University of North Carolina School
of Medicine, Chapel Hill,
North Carolina 27514, USA and
Vice President of Biomedical Affairs,
Family Health International,
PO Box 13950, Research Triangle
Park, North Carolina 27709, USA

Mr Jonathan O. Herod
Fellow in Gynaecological Oncology,
The Royal Marsden Hospital,
Fulham Road, London SW3 6JJ

Mr Andrew Hextall
Registrar in Urogynaecology, King's
College Hospital, Denmark Hill,
London SE5 9RS

Mr Richard B. Johanson
Consultant Obstetrician and
Gynaecologist, Academic
Department of Obstetrics and
Gynaecology,
North Staffordshire Hospital,
Maternity Unit,
City General Hospital,
Newcastle Road, Stoke-on-Trent
ST4 6QG

Mr Richard Kerr-Wilson
Consultant Obstetrician and
Gynaecologist,
Cheltenham General Hospital,
Sandford Road, Cheltenham,
Gloucester GL53 7AN

Ms Allison Laird
Managing Editor, *British Journal of
Obstetrics and Gynaecology*,
27 Sussex Place, Regent's Park,
London NW1 4RG

Professor David M. Luesley
Professor of Gynaecological
Oncology,
City Hospital, Dudley Road,
Birmingham B18 7QH

Dr Kirstie McKenzie-McHarg
Trials Co-ordinator/Researcher,
National Perinatal Epidemiology
Unit, Radcliffe Infirmary,
Woodstock Road,
Oxford OX2 6HE

Professor P.M. Shaughn O'Brien
Professor and Head of Academic
Department of Obstetrics and
Gynaecology,
North Staffordshire Hospital,
Maternity Unit,
City General Hospital,
Newcastle Road, Stoke-on-Trent
ST4 6QG

Dr Gillian C. Penney
Programme Co-ordinator, Scottish
Programme for Clinical Effective-
ness in Reproductive Health,
Dugald Baird Centre for Research
on Women's Health,
Aberdeen Maternity Hospital,
Cornhill Road, Aberdeen AB25 2ZL

Mr Charles W.E. Redman
Consultant Obstetrician and
Gynaecologist, Academic
Department of Obstetrics and
Gynaecology,
North Staffordshire Hospital,
Maternity Unit,
City General Hospital,
Newcastle Road, Stoke-on-Trent
ST4 6QG

Dr Paul B. Silcocks
Associate Director, Research and
Development, Trent Cancer
Registry,
Weston Park Hospital NHS Trust,
Whitham Road, Sheffield S10 2SJ

Ms Patricia C. Want
Librarian, Royal College of
Obstetricians and Gynaecologists,
27 Sussex Place, Regent's Park,
London NW1 4RG

Dr Katrina M. Wyatt
Research Fellow, Academic
Department of Obstetrics and
Gynaecology,
North Staffordshire Hospital,
Maternity Unit,
City General Hospital,
Newcastle Road, Stoke-on-Trent
ST4 6QG

Preface

We have written and published together intermittently over the past 20 years, particularly in the early part of this time when we were both with the Academic Department of Obstetrics and Gynaecology at the City Hospital, Nottingham. In that time medical research has seen many changes. The role, place and even the purpose of undertaking research has changed.

This text is written for specialists and trainees – not just medical specialists and trainees but those in all subjects related to health. Because of the nature of our posts and contacts there is a resulting emphasis on the specialist registrar trainee and many of the writers and thus the examples in the text are obstetric and gynaecological – physicians and surgeons need not feel threatened by this!

It is also true that research questions will creep into Royal College membership examinations over the next couple of years.

Whether it is the spirit of enquiry, the pursuit of an original idea or pragmatism of obtaining Membership of your College or a research degree to enable your ascent up one of the many career ladders, we that hope this text provides encouragement, insight and direction.

Fiona Broughton Pipkin
Shaughn O'Brien

1

Research and the specialist registrar

P.M. Shaughn O'Brien

Why do research?

It is now well established that specialist registrars (SpR) should, during their training, develop an understanding of research methodology. There is no better way to achieve this than to undertake research. There are, however, many motives for doing research. They include the (fairly remote) chance of making an important discovery, the enjoyment of the process of undertaking research, the hope of altering accepted management of a disease and making patients better through your own discovery and there is the buzz of working in an intellectual environment. You will note that financial reward does not appear in this list, for very good reasons, and only a few researchers (and no specialist registrars) have yet received a Nobel prize.

There are other reasons for doing research which are more pragmatic. There will, for instance, be questions on research methodology in future Membership examinations of the Royal Colleges. Research is now a requirement in all subspecialty training programmes. It is usually easier to obtain a consultant post with an MD ('awarded' not 'in preparation') and those who have demonstrated their ability to be 'doers' and 'completer/finishers' will be rewarded with a greater choice of consultant posts. It is rare to be appointed even to non-academic posts in teaching hospitals or other major centres without a higher degree in addition to Membership of a Royal College. Few consultants are now appointed to their first choice of post without having published papers.

Of course, any trainee wishing ultimately to pursue a career in academic medicine will need to obtain a postgraduate research degree such as an MD or, increasingly, a PhD.

In the 1993 report *Hospital Doctors: Training for the Future* (the Calman Report) it was clear that those responsible, at government level, for defining the training of hospital specialists were aware of the needs and opportunities for research during specialist training. It was recommended that all doctors in training should learn how to interpret and apply research findings and that specific provision should be made for those who wish to undertake research and/or prepare for an academic career.

The basic principle of the new SpR grade is that, during their specialist training, doctors should:

- be expected to develop an understanding of research methodology (and

this is why the new MRCOG examination will increasingly include questions related to audit, research papers, assessment of clinical trials and the interpretation of data)
- be encouraged to undertake research.

There are four main groups of doctors who will wish to undertake research during higher specialist training:
- The majority of doctors who undertake a period in research during higher specialist training will ultimately wish to pursue a clinical career. They will aim to complete a specialist training programme and to be awarded a Certificate of Completion of Specialist Training (CCST) giving them access to the Specialist Register. Good papers may be more appropriate than a degree for this group.
- A smaller group of doctors who intend to pursue a career in academic or research medicine will, in most cases, also wish to obtain a CCST in a recognised discipline. Although these doctors should have no less thorough clinical training than other specialist registrars, the content of their training programme, while meeting the requirements set out in the appropriate College curriculum, will have to take into account the need to develop both their research and their clinical skills. Development of educational skills will also be an important component of their training. The recently published report by Lord Dearing makes it clear that the acquisition of 'key skills' related to learning and imparting knowledge should still be a formal goal even at doctoral level.
- All subspecialty training programmes involve an important research component and it is often impossible to obtain such training posts without having undertaken research to the level of MD. These trainees may ultimately become pure clinical subspecialists or academics.
- A very small group of trainees may ultimately go into highly specialised fields of predominantly research work and very little clinical work.

What should be my research aims?

The individual's purpose in doing the research will dictate when and how it is undertaken. The goal will thus vary but publication in one way or another is essential. If research has been performed but not published then it is considered incomplete and better if not started in the first place. This is because of the waste of the researcher's and collaborator's/supervisor's time and the waste of resources. There are many ways in which research can be published:
- as a verbal presentation or poster with a published abstract (this should normally be followed by a full publication)
- as a peer-reviewed research paper
- as a higher degree thesis
- as a part of a review article
- as an electronic publication (e.g. *The Cochrane Library*).

All undergraduates should have been introduced to research at an early stage when producing a dissertation or mini-thesis in part fulfilment of the requirements for a degree. A dissertation may form part of a:

- Bachelor of Science (BSc) degree
- Master of Science (MSc)
- Bachelor of Medical Science (BMedSci)
- Master of Medical Science (MMed Sci)
- Master of Philosophy (MPhil)
- Doctor of Philosophy (PhD)
- Doctor of Medicine (MD).

The BSc, MSc and BMedSci degrees are usually taught, with a dissertation providing a proportion of the credits. MPhil is usually a research-based degree by thesis and most universities require the candidate to register for this before being 'promoted' to PhD on the basis of progress of the research and the researcher.

The PhD has previously been considered to be more scientifically oriented and the MD more clinically based research, though in my experience of examining theses there is much overlap these days. PhD theses have always been closely supervised, while MD theses were not until recently. There are historical grounds for this. Until relatively recently, the MD tended to be more of a distillation of many years' clinical experience focused on a particular topic, rather than a structured investigation. This has changed. All research theses are now considered as research training and all are formally supervised, which is appropriate.

In general, research undertaken by non-medical graduates would be as part of an MPhil or PhD and usually requires three to four years' single-minded study for completion. Medical specialist trainees would do a PhD or MD. A PhD is more internationally accepted as a research higher degree and those aspiring to an academic career at a high level would, in the present day, perhaps be well-advised to pursue this line. Furthermore, in the USA and in parts of Asia the MD is the name of the basic medical degree, which can give rise to confusion. The MD can be and often is completed in two years.

The MMed Sci degree is a developing degree particularly suited to the non-subspecialist trainee. These degrees usually contain a considerable taught element, including such subjects as:

- ethics and law
- epidemiology
- theoretical research methodology
- statistics
- medical education
- clinical effectiveness
- science and technology
- health service management.

In addition, there are specialty-specific training modules which may also be recognised for other training (but, of course, not for another degree). Examples would include recognised laparoscopic surgery training, ultrasound/imaging and so on. Finally, there is a specialty-related research dissertation and this is what usually distinguishes a Masters degree from a Diploma. This type of degree may eventually prove to be more appropriate than an MD for the non-academic trainee, in that it provides the foundation for those skills and knowledge required by the consultant of 2000 and beyond. The supervised research within this would be more than adequate to provide an understanding of research methodology as required by the time of attainment of the CCST.

What subject should I research?

The content and conduct of your research is, in theory, down to personal choice. However, it is rarely that simple. Funding must be provided for salaries and the expenses of equipment and material. It is virtually impossible to make a successful research application without research experience and a track record. In other words, you will be dependent on an established researcher or research unit. You will need a great deal of training and supervision from the outset and so the only practical way forward is to apply for a post in an established unit which will provide all of these. These posts will almost invariably be externally funded from 'soft' (grant) money. It takes time, perseverance and luck to get such money. Start planning early with your potential supervisor.

The range of research open to SpRs is enormous. It can be in clinical trials, laboratory research, basic science, epidemiology, social science, psychology, biomedical engineering and technology, imaging, screening, education, molecular medicine and so on and these can be conducted in animal research, hospital or general practice patients, healthy volunteers, computer models or indeed in libraries.

An increasing number of research units recognise detailed literature reviews and meta-analyses as fully adequate for a research thesis. Many others would think that such research is merely the starting point for genuine research. An initial literature review is always necessary to determine that an important question remains unanswered and that your new trial or study is justified from an economic (time and money) and ethical standpoint (Table 1.1).

When should I undertake research during training?

The last government introduced the requirement for a very basic understanding of research and enquiry into secondary school education at Key Stage 3 of the National Curriculum. All undergraduates should be introduced to research at an early stage. All current training in health subjects addresses research in the course of training and all medical schools allow undergradu-

Table 1.1 Some words of advice

What?	Why?
Aim for a full time post.	When you have a clinical responsibility sick patients will come first. If your post is not full time protect the research time.
Choose a subject which catches your imagination.	If you slot into a research programme and 'follow the recipe' of your supervisor, using previously collected tissue samples from the freezer, you will complete the work and obtain a degree but may never become excited about the research. However, if you rely solely on your own inspiration you may never even get started.
Choose the research unit carefully.	A proven track record will maximise your chance of completion.
Choose your supervisor carefully.	You interview the supervisor: Is he still research active/publishing? What is his prior 'hit rate' with theses? Can you get on together?

Discuss ownership of the project and authorship at the outset.

MRC, Regional or College Research Training Fellowships and similar are the best deal and are most prestigious.

ates to take a research-based intercalated BSc degree, usually taken by those identified as 'high flyers'. In some medical schools there is a compulsory year during which a research project is undertaken, leading to a Bachelor's degree. These are starting points.

The introduction of Calman training has involved major changes which are still evolving. One cannot thus be certain when is the most appropriate time to undertake research. It is to be hoped that the stage will not be reached where the Membership examination and an MD will be a prerequisite to obtaining the first SpR post.

There are great advantages to undertaking research as a senior house officer. There are fewer clinical or surgical skills to lose, the step up the career path occurs earlier, the research ethic becomes established and so one's approach to using evidence in patient management will develop earlier. On the down side, it may limit what research topic may be undertaken because of the limited amount of clinical experience accumulated and the maturity of clinical decision making.

Most trainees will take time out for research, having obtained a formal training post with a National Training Number (NTN) and retaining the NTN

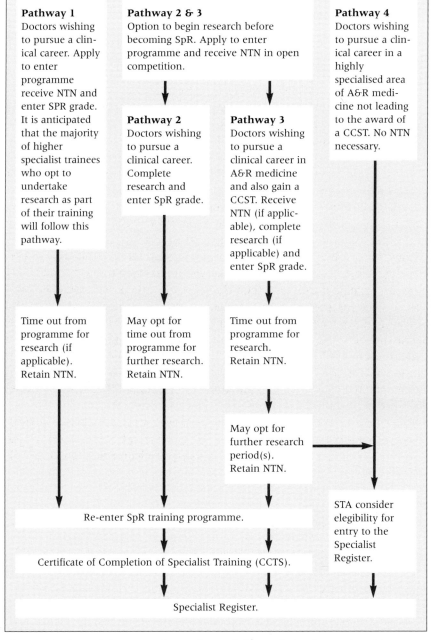

Figure 1.1 Potential career pathways for specialist medical trainees who wish to undertake a period of research time (by permission of the Department of Health and Professor John Temple, Special Advisor to the Chief Medical Officer)

during the research period. One year of research training is recognised towards CCST, but more than this is not. While you take your time out, the post is filled by a long-term locum appointment for training (LAT) or a visiting SpR.

While in the research post, prior to obtaining an NTN, that trainee is eligible to apply for a training number (in competition) and to continue in research with their number. Any moves into or out of posts that are related to NTN posts must have the approval of the Postgraduate Dean. Moves between Deaneries is possible. Those wishing to undertake an academic career are advised to do their research within a lecturer post which has full SpR recognition leading to CCST. As you will be training in clinical and academic medicine with less time for each you will be required to take longer to achieve the CCST – this is not necessarily disadvantageous in any way. Some who have begun research as an SHO may re-enter research again by taking time out during the SpR programme (Figure 1.1).

The arrangements for specialist training have, at least in theory, been designed to be as flexible as possible for doctors wishing to pursue many career pathways: from those following a purely clinical career but who need to have the research know-how to interpret research data and use this in their decision making when they treat patients, to those wishing to undertake research in combination with their clinical work. Others will wish to follow a career which is predominantly academic with a balance of clinical work, teaching and research. A very small group will become so taken by their research that they abandon clinical work altogether in favour of research. You will probably not know to which of the categories you belong. You cannot really know until you are well into your research training. The contribution of all of these people is vital to the future of individual specialties and indeed to the NHS.

The chapters which follow in this book deal with many of the subjects above and more in great detail. They will provide valuable support for the novice and a source of inspiration for budding academics and thinking clinicians.

Further reading

Royal College of Physicians Academic Research Group (1997) *Guidelines for Clinicians Entering Research*. London: RCP

Temple, J. (1998) *A Guide to Specialist Registrar Training*. London: Department of Health

2

Time management

Charles W.E. Redman

Introduction

Involvement in research, whether as a research fellow or in a clinical post, provides the opportunity of learning a variety of different skills and disciplines. Many of these will have a wider application in one's clinical career and none more so than time management. Time is said to be a linear parameter, but during research its passage can defy physics. At first it may stretch out into the future almost infinitely and pass so slowly that the challenge is how to fill it. Then, ever faster, as in free fall sky diving, the deadlines rush towards you. The key to success, be it in research or in a medical career generally, is to manage time. A number of excellent texts describe classic time management but to save your time, this short chapter summarises their key points.

'Doing' is not necessarily achieving and this is particularly so in research. 'Research is to see what everybody else has seen, and to think what nobody else has thought' (Albert Szent-Györgyi, discoverer of vitamin C and Nobel Prize winner). Thinking needs time which has to be set aside, not only for thought but also for planning.

Planning

At the outset of any project or task there are three key questions that you need to address. These are:

- How much time do I have?
- What do I have to do?
- How am I going to do it?

The first question is usually the easiest as this is often defined for you either in terms of funding or stated deadlines. It can relate to a longer period, such as the duration of a research fellowship, or simply to the forthcoming week or day. It is important to have determined at the outset how much time is to be spent working rather than in other important areas of your life. It is also prudent to make your plans with time to spare, as there are inevitably interruptions or unscheduled hitches that would otherwise compromise your plans. In short, be realistic and not over-ambitious.

The second question is not so straightforward, as there are often supplementary ones such as whether you need or should be doing it anyway. But if this is something you need to do then it becomes a 'goal'. At any one time you may have a number of goals and the process for achieving them can be broken down into smaller, individual, tasks.

The third item is about realising these tasks within the timescale you have set and requires drawing up a timetable.

Setting goals

A goal defines what you want to achieve, be it in life generally or professionally. In the context of research it can be obtaining a thesis, a grant, a publication or whatever it is you are wanting as the return for your investment of time and effort.

If you are taking a long-term strategic view, such as 'what do I want in life?' or 'what am I aiming to achieve in the next two years?', you will identify a number of major goals which you then work towards. To this end you will probably identify a number of minor goals to aim for on the way, as you move towards your major goal. Clearly there are different orders of goals depending on the time-frame in which you are working. In other words, as you write your thesis, a major goal, you need to have the introduction written by next month, a minor goal.

You will usually have a number of different goals which are all making demands on your time and often threatening to outstrip it. It is unrealistic to have too many major goals, as you will be at risk of fighting on too many fronts and winning nothing. So it is also vital that before you launch into the fray you have decided which goals are the most important and planned accordingly.

In practical terms it is a good idea to sit down every so often to review what your goals are and how you are progressing. This may be every year, or more often, but you must have in mind your priorities as this will determine how you spend your time.

Tasking

The individual steps towards reaching goals are tasks. The relationship between major goals, minor goals and tasks is hierarchical and is best illustrated by the tree analogy (Figure 2.1) in which:
- the trunk = major goal
- the branches = minor goals
- the leaves = tasks.

The key point about this concept is that large pieces of work can be broken down into smaller manageable parts. People are often daunted by the enormity of certain projects, but this can be overcome by breaking them down into their component parts. In other words: 'Q: How do you eat an elephant? A: In many meals and in little pieces!'

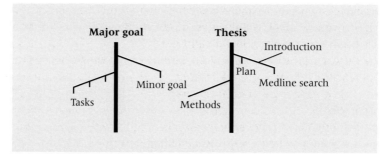

Figure 2.1 The relationship between major goals, minor goals and tasks

Prioritisation

Having defined your goals and identified the component tasks that are going to need to be achieved within a given time, say the next week, you will have a list of items all competing for your time. If it is unlikely that you will be able to do all these tasks, you will have to decide what to do, what not to do and what you may do if there is time. This is prioritisation.

One method is to triage the tasks into one of three categories, namely:

- essential
- important
- less important.

That bit is easy but it is how you do it that counts. It could be done purely on the basis of deadlines or whether the tasks are important to you, to others or to no-one in particular. Whatever method you use, the important thing is that the jobs to do are prioritised so that the important tasks get done, even if this has to be at the expense of less important ones. If you do not prioritise the reverse often happens.

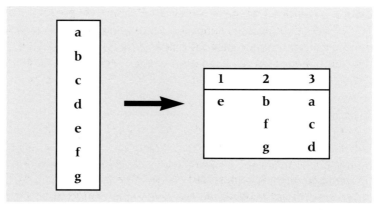

Figure 2.2 Prioritise goals and tasks. Make a list of the tasks to do and then sort them into priority categories

This exercise is worth doing on a weekly basis as you work out what needs doing in the time available. Make a list of what has to be done and prioritise each task. Having made this list, it can be helpful to rewrite the list using a column for each priority (Figure 2.2). Produce your timetable of available time and allocate time to each task in order of priority. If you run out of available time, so be it. If you do not have enough time to achieve the top priority tasks then you have a problem. Either your prior planning has been poor or you have an unrealistic number of major goals and something has to go. If the balloon is sinking you have to throw something out!

Timetabling

Much of the above is about timetabling but it is worth making some additional points. Firstly, be realistic about how long something will take. It is counterproductive to produce an over-ambitious plan for the week and doom yourself to failure at the outset. In addition, be realistic about what should be done in the time available; do not try making a silk purse out of a sow's ear and do what you can. Stop doing it when it is good enough. It is pointless striving for perfection and going well down the path of diminishing returns when that time could have been better used for something else.

When making out your timetable leave enough time to eat, sleep, relax and enjoy yourself. Furthermore, if at any stage you achieve targets ahead of schedule, do not necessarily rush on to the next one but take the advantage of this lull to reward yourself with a break and do something different.

Deadlines

Much of time management is about working to deadlines. In research, most deadlines concern dates of submission for grants or abstracts when plenty of notice is available. The cardinal rule about deadlines is that you should not break them and should do everything in your power to meet them. If the deadline is set by others, you have to decide at the outset whether the task is worth doing and if the deadline is reasonable. There is no point in committing yourself to something that cannot be done in the time available; instead, you should decline it or renegotiate the deadline. To do otherwise compounds the felony and only puts your head on the block. However, once you have accepted a deadline, be it set by yourself or others, then you must work to it.

Saving time

While planning is an essential part of making the best use of time, working efficiently is also important. There are a number of skills that can help significantly. Learn to say 'No' and avoid doing somebody else's work. Wherever possible delegate tasks to others but do so appropriately as failure will rebound on you. Master information technology skills, including how to type. Direct input of data into computer spreadsheets or databases is a vital skill and, increasingly, a portable 'lap top' is essential. Nonetheless, despite the acquisition of these other skills, planning remains pivotal. Without planning, your work will be entropic. One example of the efficient use of time is, in the course of presenting your work at meetings, to work on the relevant papers at this time. It is much easier to do this while the ideas and responses of other participants are fresh in your mind. All too often work is presented and the paper is written much later.

Wasting time

'I would I could stand at a busy corner, hat in hand, and beg people to throw me all their wasted hours' (Bernard Berenson). Whatever gains you make by working more efficiently can be dissipated by the time you waste. It is sometimes worth making a log of how you spend your time, so you can analyse how it is actually spent. This can help you to identify those tasks that you could have avoided or delegated to others, as well as suggest ways in which you could work better. Why go to the library on three separate occasions when you could have done what you wanted to do in a single visit?

One of the greatest hindrances to getting things done is procrastination. This often occurs because the task in question is seen as large and daunting while other smaller, but less important, tasks can be easily done in the time available. You must avoid this. Breaking the larger tasks down into smaller parts which can be tackled in the time available is the key.

Delegation

This is a potentially important way of saving time. When facing a task it is advised that you should decide (a) if it needs doing and (b) should *you* be doing it? Whenever possible avoid carrying out a task that could or should be carried out by someone else; this can be done in one of three ways:

- refusal
- palming off
- delegation.

If you have no vested interest in the task and it is not your responsibility, then simply say 'no'. However, it may be easier to 'palm off' the task to someone else. The difference between this and delegation is that when you palm off a task you are indifferent to the outcome, whereas when you delegate you care. In other words, although delegation can save time, you retain responsibility. Consequently, it is in your best interests to ensure that your delegation is carried out appropriately, i.e. the right task for the right person with adequate explanation and supervision. Poor delegation will result in your having to undo what has been done, or doing the job yourself, and be counterproductive. It is important to recognise that, initially, delegation may be a time-consuming activity as you ensure that things are done properly. The saying 'if you want a job doing properly, do it yourself' is not necessarily the case when delegation works. Incentives, such as co-authorship or acknowledgement, promote successful delegation and failure to give due recognition will jeopardise future success.

Delegation implies the handing-down of a task, whereas most junior researchers are already in the basement. However, there is often scope for collaboration in which tasks can be shared. Indeed, an increasing feature of modern clinical research is the formation of teams comprised of individuals providing different skills, e.g. clinicians, biochemists, statisticians, data managers, etc. Nonetheless, whether you delegate or collaborate the process has to be thought through and not simply be allowed to happen, lest it become counterproductive.

Hiding

There are many detractors from study:

- bleeps
- supervisors
- NHS colleagues saying 'We're short, come and help out with the clinic'
- patients
- colleagues, friends and family.

One way of ring-fencing your time is to identify a location which is protected from the outside world. This could be a study, a carrel in the library, a train or an aeroplane.

Final comments

Time spent in research can be very rewarding, providing the opportunity to learn a variety of skills which often have wider application. The time available for research is limited for most doctors and it is a precious resource which to some degree can be expanded or lost depending on its use. 'Gather ye rosebuds while ye may, Old Time is still a-flying' (Robert Herrick, 1591–1674, *To the Virgins, to Make Much of Time*).

## 3

Basic computer skills, word processing, databases, spreadsheets and presentation packages

Robin Burr

Introduction

The advent of the electronic age has revolutionised the way we work and communicate. Rapid and continuing advances in this technology have given the individual user the type of processing power in a personal computer (PC) that previously was only available in large mainframe machines. The PC has provided the scientific worker and clinician with an invaluable tool for their work. Not only have previously laborious work practices been transformed, but the PC has enabled entirely new ways of working to be developed. Possibly the most useful advance for the research worker is the electronic transfer of information between computers, both locally and globally over the Internet. The fierce competition in the PC market has ensured that a relatively powerful combination of hardware and software is an inexpensive option that all researchers should be using to enhance the quality of their efforts. This chapter is intentionally basic; most advances beyond this are obtained from practical experience with the programs, together with informal advice from more experienced users or practical courses run by the university.

Basic computing skills

In the days of DOS (disk operating system), the PC user had to learn a complex series of commands to operate the computer, followed by another set of commands for each application program used. Every program would have its own individual set of commands which would often be very different from any other program with similar functions. These commands would have to be typed in at a command line with reference to a bulky manual. Thankfully for those of us with limited keyboard skills but reasonable hand–eye co-ordination, the advent of the Windows® operating system provided a graphical interface together with a mouse (a pointing device controlling an on-screen cursor and other functions) to provide a more simple means of interacting with the computer. On-screen help became available and the manuals started to become thinner. However, there were still large differences in the way in which the various application programs interfaced with the user, with very few being intuitive.

Users of Apple Macintosh® computers have long had the benefit of a common 'look and feel' to a wide variety of programs, and this is a more recent phenomenon with computers running Windows 95®. The latest versions of the major software suites of programs now all have a common look and feel between the individual programs, although they are only common to the individual manufacturer.

As Microsoft Windows® is the most widely used operating system in the world, this chapter will concentrate on software that runs on this operating system. When buying a new PC in 1999 it will usually be preloaded with Windows 98® as the operating system and will often also include one or other of the major software suites of application programs, such as Microsoft Office®.

Currently, all the mainstream software packages have comprehensive on-screen help which enables the first-time user to achieve a decent level of proficiency in a relatively short time. This online help varies from the vital to the extremely irritating, according to the level of expertise of the user, although most can be switched off. Most software manuals are now bordering on the anorexic and consequently there is now a large market for independent books explaining how to use the main software packages. Examples include the *Que Quick Reference* series and the *For Dummies* series, covering all the major software programs.

Microsoft itself has the lion's share of the applications software market with its Office® suite, followed by IBM's Lotus Smartsuite® and Corel's Wordperfect® Suite. All these software suites contain a word processor, spreadsheet, database and presentation package, as well as other programs, such as a personal information organiser.

To the average individual there are no significant differences between these packages, in that the ability of each program is well in excess of the needs of the average user. It has been estimated that, for 80% of the time, the average user only uses 20% of the functions in a software program. So the choice of which software programs to use depends on variables such as which particular software was sold with the computer or which screen appearance is preferable or which software is used at work, in the department or in the university as a whole. All the major programs will be able to read the data files created by their competitors and most provide a relatively easy means of converting other files into their own format.

Word processing

Possibly the most valuable program for the average user is the word processing program and this program is the reason many people buy a PC. The advantages of word processing programs are so overwhelming that they have virtually completely replaced the typewriter. One major advantage of the PC is that work can be stored on a disk (either floppy disk for transfer between computers or on the internal hard disk) for future amendments and editing. Any number of copies, in a variety of formats, can be printed without having to retype a single word. If amendments are necessary, these can very easily be incorporated without having to retype the whole document. The same piece of work can also be printed on a wide variety of printers, both colour and black-and-white. The creator has total control over the final appearance of the printed work and can easily preview a variety of different versions on-screen prior to printing the final version. In fact, the latest versions of the major word processors are so sophisticated that there is a large overlap with the functions usually found in the highly sophisticated desktop publishing programs. The major word processing packages are Microsoft's Word for Windows®, IBM's Lotus Word Pro® and Corel's Wordperfect®. Essentially, there are no significant differences in functionality between these programs and personal preference is the best reason for preferring one over another.

Other functions now standard that are invaluable for producing a professional quality document include the spell-checker, format checker and thesaurus. Although the standard spell-checker is unlikely to contain specialised and technical words, these can be added to a user dictionary or even bought as additions to the main program. The ability to create tables of contents and indexes, together with the creation of graphs, tables and graphics including equations are functions available in all the major programs. All the main word processing programs now provide integration with the other programs in the suite, so that graphs, spreadsheets and databases can be readily incorporated into a document with the advantage that, when the original is changed, the copy in the document is automatically updated. Mail merging is a very useful function when a standard letter has to be sent to a large number of people – this is commonly seen in the vast and increasing amount of 'personalised' junk mail delivered by the postal service.

As increasing numbers of publications are now multi-authored, a fast and convenient means of reviewing the article is afforded by emailing the file to all the authors, either over a local area network (such as a university network) or globally via the Internet. The advantage of this means of communication over posted or faxed versions is that the second author can make corrections and amendments directly to the original document, prior to emailing it back to the first author.

For the researcher with references to organise, a reference manager program can save an enormous amount of time. Although there is no shortcut to the time-consuming chore of entering the individual references into the program, its value when formatting the final paper soon becomes apparent. For an additional expense, this type of program can also import references electronically from CD-ROMs or via Medline. All these programs can produce a bibliography in a wide variety of standard formats required by the major journals in a fraction of the time it would take to do the same process manually. Should the style of the bibliography need changing, for example, for submission to a second journal, then this can easily be accomplished without having to retype any of the original document. Of course, the database of references created can be used for any number of documents in the future.

For those who find typing (even the two-finger method used by this author) difficult and slow, there are now voice recognition programs that translate the spoken word into the typewritten version. Although attractive at first sight, limitations with this type of program still require a fair amount of typing to correct errors, even after extensive training of the program. Ultimately, however, this type of program will become the standard method of interfacing with a PC. In the meantime, a short course on typing skills may, for most of us, prove to be more valuable than the detailed anatomy of the mid-brain!

Databases

Although word processing is probably the commonest use for a PC, their real value is in data processing. The PC is essentially a simple calculator and is ideal for processing any form of data, both numerical and text. A notebook computer provides a method of collecting data in the field and a network of PCs allows many users to enter data into the same database.

A database provides a standardised method of entering data and each data field can be validated, in that only one of a set number of responses can be entered into that field. The database can readily be updated and amendments easily made if necessary. Also, an entry for each field can be required by the program to avoid loss of data – both major advantages over a paper-based method of data collection. Storing data on a PC provides a very compact method of storage when compared with the paper-based method, although a secure means of backing up or making a copy of the data is vital. Remember, researchers have lost whole PhD theses in computer crashes or faulty floppy disks. A 'belt and braces' approach is strongly recommended to back up all important data – both electronically and paper-based.

The real strength of databases is evident when the collected data are then collated and processed. Performing searches on a computerised database is infinitely quicker and more accurate than hand-searching a mass of paper forms. Not only that, but complex searches can easily be created and saved for later reuse. The subset of data thus found can then be saved into a new file or imported into a spreadsheet for statistical analysis. New data fields can be created from performing calculations on existing data fields and then incorporated into searches.

Database programs may either be 'flat file' or 'relational' in nature. Flat file databases store each record as an individual item so that any field common to another record must be retyped into each and every record. This can be very time-consuming where there are large amounts of data common to each record, such as where one patient has a number of observations made at different times – the patient details would have to be entered into each record of the observations at every event. A relational database stores the data in several separate files that are cross-referenced. In the above example, the patient data would only be entered once into a separate file then cross-referenced with the observational data files as required. Although this would require slightly more time to create, it allows for a very efficient and powerful database to be developed. Each file created can be cross-referenced or linked to any other database file and can thus be reused any number of times. When considering using a database, the additional effort required in creating a relational database will provide its own rewards when using the database both to enter and, later, to process the data. The latest versions of the major database programs all provide ready-made templates and help routines for creating quite complex databases without needing any knowledge of programming.

Most database programs will provide a number of means of producing an output. This may take the form of a printed report, a graph or a file incorporated into another document. Again, the major programs all provide a great deal of help in producing whatever type of output is required.

Designing a database is relatively easy but it needs careful consideration, together with a number of 'dry runs' prior to the main data entry, as it can be difficult to reconfigure the database later, when it already contains a quantity of precious data. It is also important to consider the end use of data because there is very little point in having collected a quantity of data that cannot later be processed in a useful and meaningful manner. For example, many maternity databases are very easy to enter data into but have limited or no facility for the non-standard searches that a researcher would want to perform. As there will usually be a need for statistical analysis of the data collected it is well worth considering the type of data output that the statistical program or a statistician will require when designing the database. Advice of this nature should be sought during the design phase of the research protocol and its database.

Spreadsheets

A spreadsheet program provides a powerful means of manipulating data, ranging from simple calculations to complex statistical and financial functions. Multiple calculations can be performed on the dataset on a 'what if' basis, that is, determining the effect of changing one piece of data on the rest of the dataset without losing any of the original data. This is particularly, although not exclusively, valuable in financial spreadsheets.

A spreadsheet consists of a number of cells labelled alphabetically along the columns and numerically down the rows. Each cell can contain any type of data, both numerical and text or formulae. The major programs come with a wide and comprehensive range of formulae that include means of manipulating financial, mathematical, statistical, trigonometrical, calendar, logical and text-based data, among others. Data can readily be sorted in any order on any particular type of criteria – both alphabetical and numerical.

Spreadsheets will also include database-type functions which are particularly useful for managing small volumes of data, although for large amounts of data a specific database program is more suitable. Most spreadsheets will allow data to be imported or directly linked to data within a database –

although usually only from the database within the same manufacturer's suite of programs.

All spreadsheets come with extensive and powerful charting capabilities for producing professional quality documents – either directly from the program itself or when imported into or linked to a word processor file. A colour ink-jet or laser printer will demonstrate the impressive quality of charting output from a spreadsheet program.

Statistical analysis has always been a strong point of the spreadsheet program and is usually an integral part of any research project. Depending on the nature and complexity of the analysis (and the ability of the researcher) the spreadsheet program may provide all the required functions. Even if this is all that is required for data analysis it is wise to seek the advice of a statistician prior to collecting and analysing data. For larger datasets and complex analyses a statistical package may be a better means of analysing the data. In this case, discussion with the statistician using the statistical program will ensure not only that the correct data are collected but also that the output from the spreadsheet program is compatible with the statistical program.

The most recent versions of spreadsheet programs offer '3D spreadsheets'. In this situation a number of separate spreadsheets can be interlinked so that calculations can be performed on cells across a number of different spreadsheets, with the results exported to or saved in a separate spreadsheet.

Although initially the program that made the PC a valuable tool, spreadsheets have had a reputation for being difficult to use. This has largely, although not entirely, been addressed by the software manufacturers, who have included a number of templates and help routines for creating new spreadsheets. Spreadsheets, columns and ranges of data can now be labelled with more intuitive names which can, in turn, be used in calculations and formulae.

Presentation packages

All researchers will have to present their work at some point, and whether this is an in-house talk or a presentation at an international meeting, good quality visual aids are essential for getting the message across clearly. The advantage of using a PC to produce these visual aids is that the creator has total control over the content and appearance of the work. Not only that, but the original files are stored on disk and can be reused any number of times and to produce any number and type of output.

The simplest and cheapest means of providing a visual aid is to photocopy the printed output from a word processor on to acetates, for use with an overhead projector. Although well-considered use of fonts and arrangement can produce a clear overhead, this method is rather limited. Using a colour ink-jet printer with the appropriate acetates will allow colour overheads to be produced directly from the PC at short notice. Virtually all auditoriums, however small, will have an overhead projector, which is relatively simple technology. Whatever the primary means of presenting it may be worth having a (colour) copy on overheads as a backup.

A specialised presentation package will provide a more comprehensive method of producing a presentation in a number of formats. This provides total control over all the aspects of producing a slide and will create a common appearance to all the slides in the presentation. A variety of graphics is provided with the program or can be imported from clip-art or created with the aid of a scanner. Many will also import photographs from a Photo CD-ROM. In addition, most have a comprehensive range of graphics to produce organisational and flowcharts. All the programs will have templates and help routines for the relatively easy creation of a presentation.

A more professional appearance is gained when using 35-mm slides, using single or dual projection facilities. Any of the presentation packages in the major software suites will produce an output suitable for creating 35-mm slides. As the equipment for creating slides from a presentation package is expensive, it is usually found only in professional bureaux or in larger audio-visual departments. The files created can be sent by disk or via a modem to a bureau for creating slides. Each frame in the presentation can have a text note attached and the slide and note can be printed out on the same paper page as the speaker's notes. A number of slides can be printed out on each page to be used as audience handouts. The slides created for a presentation can be viewed on-screen and the timings of the accompanying talk can be checked and refined. However, once created as 35-mm slides, it is expensive to correct errors or add extra slides. Although it is possible to extract slides from a variety of different presentations to create a new presentation with its own look, this new presentation would again have to be turned into 35-mm slides with the time and expense this would incur. The most widely used program for creating 35-mm slides is Microsoft Powerpoint® and as this is often the program that audiovisual departments use it is convenient to create the presentation in this format to avoid problems with file compatibility.

All the presentation packages will produce a screen show of slides, with control over the timing and nature of transitions between individual slides. A means of demonstrating this directly to the audience produces a very slick and professional presentation. Notebook computers have a port to allow connection to an external monitor and this can also be used to connect to a number of devices suitable for viewing by an audience. Such devices include LCD panels, which are placed over an overhead projector, and video projectors. Both are portable but expensive and, as with any technology, prone to equipment failure. However, where available, this form of output allows use of both moving text and images on the individual slide together with a sound output if connected to the auditorium sound system. As the use of PCs becomes ever more widespread and the equipment levels in auditoriums improve, this will become the optimal and probably standard means of giving a presentation.

With an eye to the developing potential of the Internet, all the major programs will produce output suitable for publication to the World Wide Web.

How to buy a PC

First considerations
- What do I want the computer for in the future?
- How much can I afford to spend?
- Where should I buy from?

What will I want the computer to do in the future?
This is a difficult question to answer today. Usually one's requirements increase in line with one's knowledge of the computer; thus, try to buy a computer that is either (a) in excess of today's requirements or (b) that can be upgraded at a later date. Also remember that changes in the operating systems (for example, Windows 98®) and software packages almost always put an increased demand on the hardware. It is said that you can never have too much of anything to do with the hardware side of computers – if you can afford it! Currently a PC with a Pentium II® processor and at least 32 MB of RAM is the 'entry level' model, although this changes very quickly. A browse through the PC magazines will provide an up-to-date version of what the industry is currently selling as the entry level model.

How much can I afford to spend?
As always this is the limiting factor in buying a computer. In calculating your budget remember to include the costs of any software and consumables (for example, disks, paper, ink cartridges, etc.). Many companies offer bundles of specific hardware and software that appear similar – look at the fine details and decide which package meets your needs closest. Some companies offer interest-free credit schemes from time to time – very worthwhile as long as the bundle specified meets your requirements. On a limited budget it is a good idea to spend the larger amount of money, in the first instance, on the parts of the system that cannot be upgraded or are difficult to upgrade at a later (richer!) time. Remember the value of buying using a credit card for purchases over £100 in terms of the financial protection if the goods are not delivered.

Where should I buy from?
There is now a wide range of retail outlets for computers, ranging from non-specialised high-street shops to very specialised computer dealers. Mail order forms a large part of computer sales, and it is also possible to hire computer systems.

Non-specialised high-street shops may offer good deals on specific systems, but changing the specifications to suit your requirements may not be possible. Also, it would be unreasonable to expect to get the same expert advice there as you would in a specialised computer shop. The latter, besides offering better advice, tends to have a wider variety of computers available and should be able to tailor a machine to fit your requirements. A local shop is not only convenient to buy from, but also to return the goods for repair or upgrade. However, prices tend to be higher from a shop (in view of their overheads, etc.) than from mail order companies. Advice on a system to suit you (as opposed to the salesman!) may or may not be available from mail order companies – but if you know what you want they do offer cost-savings, and will usually configure a machine to your specific requirements.

Many universities will allow students registered for higher degrees to buy software through the CHEST, which is considerably cheaper than buying on the open market. Additionally, computer hardware and software used for research purposes may be tax exempt.

All PCs will have at least a one-year warranty on a return to base (RTB) basis, whereby it is your responsibility and cost to return the faulty machine to the vendor. Some companies provide an on-site service whereby a technician will come out to fix the PC, although there is a cost factor to consider – this may be 'built in' to the price of the PC. Independent support companies exist to provide this service, again at a cost. Some vendors offer 'extended warranties', for a price, for a number of years after the initial warranty period has expired. The value of these depends on the value of having your PC available and functioning at all times. For the average user, who has been clever enough to back up their data, a short time when the machine is returned to the vendor or even to a local shop for repair is an acceptable cheap(er) option. Bear in mind that there are very few parts that can go wrong – the most common being the hard disk, as it has moving parts, and the monitor.

Monitors

The standard monitor that comes with most PC compatibles is a 14-inch version: adequate for most tasks, but if you intend to spend a long time staring at it a 15-inch monitor usually offers a clearer picture – but at increased cost. If you are planning to do a great deal of desktop publishing or CAD work then a 17-inch monitor may be more appropriate. It is worth considering carefully as not all monitors are the same, although it is an easy upgrade in the future and easy to replace should it cease to function.

Printers

The range includes dot-matrix, ink-jet and laser printers. Dot-matrix are the cheapest, but give the lowest quality printout and tend to be noisy and slow. Ink-jet printers offer almost laser quality printout, are quiet and can also print in colour. Printing times tend to be slow, especially for colour. Laser printers offer the highest quality printout, but are more expensive to buy and run. Colour printing lasers are very expensive. Many printers are sold with a computer as part of a bundle. Most of the brand leaders' products differ little in the quality or speed of printing.

Software

Software is an important part of the system, often not considered in advance. Decide what it is that you want the software to do for you, then which particular package meets those needs, then check that the hardware will run that package and, finally, find the money to buy it. Often, as with printers, a software package may be included with the computer. However, the benefits of a 'free £1000-worth of software' bundle may be less than expected if you never use any of this software.

Fax–modems

To send and receive faxes or to access online information such as the Internet, a fax–modem is required. These are either internal (they fit inside the machine) – cheaper – or external – more expensive but with indicator lights to tell you if and how they are working. The standard (currently) speed is 30 600 bps, although 56 000 bps modems are available. The faster the modem, the shorter the online time and the smaller the telephone bill. Most modems are sold with the software necessary to run them.

Backup devices

In an ideal world these would not be necessary, but to safeguard the contents of your hard disk some form of backup is a good idea. This can be to floppy disks, but more commonly and conveniently to a tape-streamer. Backups can be automated to save the whole contents of the hard disk to tape and run at a convenient time (for example, the middle of the night): a worthwhile form of insurance whose true value only becomes apparent when disaster strikes.

Finally

Remember that, as a result of the speed of change in the computer world, anything that you buy is almost immediately obsolete. This should not be entirely depressing – as long as the system that you have bought suits your needs then it is the right computer for you.

Conclusion

This chapter has endeavoured to provide the non-computer user with an outline of the value of a modern PC with a suite of application software. The various software suites have not been described in detail as their main functions are essentially identical, with the differences being largely cosmetic. Detailed help on using the multitude of functions in each program is available on-screen, in the supplied manual or in commercially available guide books.

The particular software suite used is less important than actually having access to a PC and software packages to maximise the efforts of the individual researcher and enhance the end results of their efforts.

Glossary

Application A specific task, for example stock control, for which a computerised solution exists.

ascii American Standard Code for Information Interchange. A code for relating a (binary) number to an alphanumeric character. The number is called the ascii code.

Background Refers to a non-interactive process running on a computer while the user is using another interactive process.

Backup Copying of files to a storage medium for safekeeping in the event of damage to the original.

Backward compatible A program is backward compatible if it can use files from an older version of itself. For a file saved in the program to be backward compatible, it must be possible to open the file in a previous version of the program.

Boot To start up a computer system.

Bubble-jet printer A printer which creates the character by squirting tiny ink droplets on to the paper. The quality is better than dot-matrix printers and usually almost, but not quite, as good as laser printers.

CD-ROM Compact Disk–Read Only Memory. A CD-ROM is any compact disk which contains computer data. These disks can store huge amounts of data (up to 640 megabytes). If there are large amounts of data on a CD-ROM, then it is usually impractical to copy the data on to the hard disk; in this case, you must insert the disk whenever you want to use the data. The ROM simply means that you cannot save information on to these disks. CD-ROM may also refer to the drive used to read these disks.

Character A single letter (A–Z), digit (0–9), special symbol (,.?≤≥, etc.) or code used to control a device.

CHEST Combined Higher Education

Software Team, organises the bulk purchase and special deals of software for the academic sector.

Chip A piece of semiconductor material containing electronic circuitry.

Circuit A collection of electrical elements through which electricity flows.

Code The statements, either in compiled or text form, which make a program.

Command A user instruction to the computer, usually given via the keyboard, but sometimes via a mouse or other pointing device. It can be a word or character that causes the computer to perform a specific action.

Compatibility The ability of a program, device or component to be used on more than one type of computer.

Computer network A set of interconnected computer systems, terminals and communications equipment.

Configuration The equipment making up a particular computer system, or the initialisation commands given to a system before running an application.

CPU Central Processing Unit. Electronic components in a computer that control the transfer of data and perform logical and arithmetic operations.

Crash A catastrophic failure of a computer program, often owing to faulty logic in the program. The system will require a reboot to be able to function.

Cursor A movable, blinking bar of light on a visual display unit (VDU) screen marking the next character entry or change.

Cursor key Key used to move the cursor around the screen. Usually identified by an arrow on the key face.

Data Facts, numbers, letters and symbols stored in a computer.

Database A collection of organised data to be used for an application, for example personnel information.

Device A piece of hardware that performs some specific function. Input devices, for example keyboards, get data into the computer. Output devices, for example printers, get data out of the computer. Some devices are both input and output, for example floppy disks.

Disk A thin flat circular plate coated with magnetic material and used to store data. Hard disks are rigid while floppy disks are not (although they may be housed in a rigid case, as are 3.5-inch floppies). Floppy disks come in one of two sizes – 5.25 inches (now largely obsolete) or 3.5 inches in diameter. Hard disks hold much more information than floppy disks, but generally cannot be moved from the computer as can floppy disks.

Diskette A term sometimes used to refer to a floppy disk.

DOS Disk Operating System. DOS was the standard operating system for PCs before Windows was created. It required the user to type commands at a boring screen with no pictures, no sound, no mouse, no colour. As time progressed, there were some good programs written for DOS that did offer these features (pictures, sounds, etc.), but each program usually worked in its own way, and you had to know DOS to get the programs. Then Windows was invented. At first, Windows was just an add-on to DOS, but now it is the standard operating system. DOS is still included in Windows 98, although for backward compatibility.

Dot-matrix printer A printer that forms characters from a two-dimensional pattern of dots by pins striking an inked ribbon. The more dots used, the better the quality of the printing, but quality is limited to pin size.

Drive A device that holds a disk so that the computer can use the information stored on it.

Electronic mail (email) A way of sending memos or messages from one computer to another.

EPS Encapsulated postscript.

Error message A textual message displayed when the computer detects a problem.

Extended keyboard Keyboard with more keys than the standard, typewriter-like keyboard.

File A file is a long sequence of bytes which represent data. Each file has a name and an extension which are separated by a dot (period). The name, of course, identifies the file. The extension tells the computer what type of data are contained within the file. For example, a file called 'Letter to George.DOC' is a Microsoft Word DOCUMENT.

File formats

BMP BitMap Format, for example, used by 'Paintbrush';

.JPG JPEG coded files;

.PCX Paintbrush, Ventura raster screen format (which pixels where);

.RTF Rich Text Format (Microsoft);

.TIFF Tagged Image File Format;

.WAV digitised sound/sound blaster;

.WMF Windows (graphics) Meta File.

Filename The name assigned by the user to a file so that both the user and computer can read it.

Folder A folder can be thought of as a location on your hard disk or floppy disk. Folders used to be called directories/subdirectories. A folder contains files and can contain nested folders (subfolders). Folders and subfolders are used to organise your hard disk. For example, you probably already have a folder named 'My Documents' on your hard disk; you could place a subfolder named

'Work' under 'My Documents' and place all your work documents within this subfolder. This way, you can keep your work documents separate from your personal documents.

Format (verb) To format or initialise a disk to set it up ready to receive data; (noun) a computer language statement which specifies the way in which output data are printed or displayed.

Function key Special key on a keyboard.

Graphics The use of lines and shapes to display data, as opposed to using printed characters alone.

Hard copy Output in a permanent form, usually on paper.

Hardware The tangible electronic (and mechanical) devices which constitute a computer system. This includes both the computer itself and any peripherals.

Icon Any icon is a picture used to represent an object. Some example objects are: data files, program files, folders, email messages and drives. Each type of object has a different icon. That means that different types of files each have an icon representing its file type. MS Word files will have the MS Word icon; MS Excel files will have the MS Excel icon; etc.

Ink-jet printer A type of printer which prints by controlling a jet or set of jets of ink so that the required shapes are marked on to paper (see **Bubble-jet printers**).

Input Data entered into a computer.

Internet International network of networks.

JANET Joint Academic NETwork. A computer network interconnecting mainly academic users in the United Kingdom, and with links to other computer networks abroad (see Internet).

Keyboard The set of keys which

allows characters to be sent to the computer when pressed. It inputs text and commands to the computer.

Laser printer A printer that uses a laser (or sometimes light emitting diodes or LEDs) to form its characters. Works very much like a photocopier.

Lock See **Write protect**.

Magnetic tape A thin tape coated with magnetic material and stored on reels. Only sequential access to the data is possible.

Mailbase A UK-based organisation which hosts mailing lists for the UK academic community.

Mainframe A physically large computer capable of manipulating large quantities of data and of supporting a number of concurrent users.

Memory The main high-speed storage area in a computer where a program is kept while it is being run. See also RAM and ROM.

Menu A list of options from which the user selects an action to be performed by entering a letter or moving the cursor.

Microcomputer A physically small computer, usually the cheapest type of computer.

Microprocessor A single-chip CPU.

Minicomputer A computer whose physical size lies between that of a microcomputer and a mainframe. It usually has a better performance than a microcomputer.

Modem Modulator/demodulator. A device that converts computer signals (binary data) into communications signals that can be sent over telephone wires.

Monitor A television-like device used for displaying data (see VDU).

Mouse A peripheral device incorporating a ball, which is rolled around a flat surface. The movement is translated into movement of a cursor around the monitor screen.

MPEG Motion Picture Experts Group.

Multi-tasking The ability of a computer to appear to perform more than one task at a time, usually by giving small amounts of processing time to each task in turn. Also referred to as multi-programming.

Operating system A collection of programs which controls the overall operation of the computer. It performs tasks such as validating users, scheduling jobs and controlling the peripherals.

Output Response from a computer, for example visual output on a screen, printed output, files written to disk.

Package A program or group of programs developed to perform a particular task, for example statistical analysis.

Parallel An interface in which multiple wires or signals are used to carry all of the bits in a byte at once. Parallel interfaces are inherently faster than serial ones. Printers which are connected to a computer by a parallel interface are known as parallel printers.

PC (Personal Computer) A general term for a microcomputer designed for use by a single user at a time, cf. Mainframe. Most often refers to any microcomputer resembling models made by the IBM company.

Peripheral A device that is external to the CPU and main memory but connected to it electrically, for example a printer or modem.

Plotter A hard copy device designed to display graphics.

Printer A device for producing paper copies of data. See also Dot-matrix, Ink-jet, Laser printers.

Printout Refers to anything printed out by a peripheral, or any computer-generated hard copy.

Program A collection of instructions needed to solve a particular problem or to guide the computer in its operation.

Programming languages The words and symbols, along with rules for combining them, that are used to construct computer programs. Usually these languages need to be translated into machine code before the computer can understand them (see Compiler). Examples are COBOL, FORTRAN and BASIC. Languages can be high level or low level. The higher the level, the closer the language looks to English; the lower the level the closer the language looks to a list of mnemonics and numbers.

RAM Random Access Memory. Memory that can both be written to and read from. Its contents vanish when the computer is switched off. It is usually used to store the operating system, programs and their data while running.

Reboot To restart the computer.

Record A collection of related data items, for example the personnel record of an individual.

ROM Read Only Memory. Memory that can only be read from. Its contents are permanent.

Screen The display surface of a monitor, like a television tube.

Serial A method of data transmission or an interface in which individual bits are sent one after another via a single signal or connecting wire. Serial interfaces are inherently slower than parallel ones. Printers which are connected to a computer by a serial interface are known as serial printers.

Software A term meaning computer programs and data.

SPSS Statistical Package for Social Sciences – a statistical package, used by users from all disciplines.

Stand-alone system A computer system which does not rely on other systems to perform tasks but may be linked by a computer network to any other computer.

SVGA Super VGA. 800*600 screen resolution.

System The combination of hardware and software making up a computer.

System disk A hard or floppy disk which contains essential information for booting a computer.

Tape streamer An input–output device for transferring data held on magnetic tape to and from a computer.

TIFF Tagged Image File Format.

User The person who is using or operating a computer system or terminal.

User interface The set of prompts, commands, messages, etc. provided to a user to enable him/her to use a computer program or package. A command-driven interface is one where the user controls the program by typing in a sequence of commands in response to prompts. A graphical interface is one where the user controls the program by pointing at graphics (such as menus and icons) on the screen.

VGA Video Graphics Array, IBM standard. Resolution 640*480.

Virus Rogue program which can transfer itself from one disk to another, unbeknown to the owner of the receiving disk. The virus program can then be triggered into action by certain commonplace commands or actions performed by the user. Some virus programs may simply flash messages or pictures on the screen, but others may corrupt program and data files.

Window A rectangular area on the screen that contains the interface between the user and a particular program. Several windows can be open at the same time, enabling a user to run programs simultaneously. Thus a user might have a document displayed in one window, while running an application in another. Windows are usually associated with a GUI.

Word processing A system that processes text, performing functions such as paragraphing, justification, paging and printing out.

Write enable To remove write protection.

Write protect To protect a file or disk from having data written to it or removed from it.

WYSIWYG What You See Is What You Get – it is pronounced 'wizzy-wig'. It means that what you see on your screen while you edit your file looks the same as you get when you print the file. Some older word processors were not WYSIWYG, and formatting (such as bold or underline) would show up on-screen as strange codes (but look fine when printed). Today ordinary word processors are almost always WYSIWYG; however, some software for creating web pages is not yet WYSIWYG.

WWW World Wide Web.

4

A guide to the Internet

Paul W. Dimmock
and Katrina M. Wyatt

Introduction

The Internet is rapidly becoming an integral part of everyday life for the medical community as much as for everyone else. The capabilities of the Internet in assisting clinical work and medical research are enormous and include:

- rapid access to online journals, often subscription free
- instant access to detailed clinical data anywhere in the world, including high resolution photographs and graphics
- rapid communication with colleagues in multi-centre collaborations world-wide.

The Internet is also emerging as a major source for publication of medical results and has many advantages over traditional paper-based methods. Most journals and publishing houses have an Internet presence and often allow the downloading of articles and papers.

What is it?

The Internet is a network of interconnected computers on a global scale. It was originally developed by the US military and US academic institutions in the 1960s and 1970s and it is now linked to tens of millions of computers worldwide. From its base in academic and governmental organisations it has expanded and is now increasingly being used by commercial organisations and individuals. It acts as a catalyst in the fast exchange of information and communications and can be used to contact people, as well as to gather and disseminate information.

Getting connected

Aside from the obvious requirements of a computer, the other essential piece of equipment is a modem. This will allow your computer to connect to the outside world via a telephone line. If your computer is situated within a large academic, medical or commercial institution, you may only need the installation of an additional network card to your computer to access the Internet via a local network. Your local hardware technicians (or computing department) will be the best source of advice on how to connect in this situation.

Generally, home and office Internet connections involve a computer and a modem. Most modems and modern computers will have software supplied with them to allow connection to the Internet. There are also many commercial and 'free' software options available of varying degrees of sophistication.

Internet supplier

When your computer and software are ready, an Internet provider is required to act as a point of access to the Internet. This may be one of the popular commercial suppliers such as CompuServe or BT, who may waive connection fees for an introductory period and supply free software, allowing you easy access. However, all commercial suppliers will require regular monthly payments for the continuing connection. Alternatively, many large organisations, such as hospitals or universities, allow their employees to dial into their main computer network to access the Internet free of charge, or for some small fee.

CD-ROMs with auto-connection software are often found on the front of popular computing magazines and bundled with new computers. Important factors to take into account before signing up are:

- the monthly costs of connection
- the availability and level of the service provided; for example, the number of lines available to dial in on, the speed on the connections and any provision for email
- the minimum length of the contract.

It must be remembered that either way, normal (usually local rate) telephone charges will apply while your computer is connected to the Internet.

Email

Electronic mail (email) is, as its name suggests, a message typed into a computer and sent to another computer without necessarily being printed out on paper. A computer is required with appropriate software to allow access to a central computer with an email service, normally using a modem. Your email account will come in the form of an address such as bob.smith@large. computer.com. The form of the address gives some indication of where the person is: com is a commercial organisation, edu is a US academic institution, ac.uk is a UK academic institution and so on. Most Internet providers will give an email account with Internet access. The two major methods of using email are discussed below.

Personal computer-based mode

Here, a person runs software on their personal computer which contacts a service provider via a modem, logs in and downloads the email in the user's account on to their computer. An analogy could be the postal service (Internet) and a post office box (your email account on the service provider's computer) which you must unlock (with your password) to retrieve your mail (download email to your computer). There are numerous freeware, shareware and commercial email packages available, such as Eudora, Microsoft or Outlook and these can often be linked to a web browser. These can be complex to set up but your Internet service provider should give you all the help you need. All your email should then be transferred to your computer and deleted from your remote account.

Remote computer mode

This method is popular in large organisations such as universities, where all the email accounts are on one central computer. This involves logging into a remote (usually Unix) computer and then running a mail-reading program in order to read the email on the remote computer, rather than downloading it. A typical session is shown in Figure 4.1.

This particular session uses the ELM program to read, write and send email on a remote Unix computer. You will still require a computer to access the remote computer.

Advantages and disadvantages of the two modes

PC-based method
- Allows normal editing, cut/paste, spell checks, etc. as well as access, often via generic word processing packages – so there is no need to learn obscure Unix editing programs.
- Allows email editing while not connected or 'offline'.
- Allows attachments to be sent (see below).
- Can be seamlessly integrated with web browsers.

Remote Unix-based method
- Can use a 'dumb' terminal and avoid relatively expensive computer/ modem options.
- Does not need complex set-up.
- Does not handle attachments very well.
- Thoroughly embedded in the Unix operating system, which can be user surly.

Attachments

Attachments are files attached to email messages, which may be complex formatted word processed documents, spreadsheets or graphics. These files can be transferred and downloaded as part of a normal text-based email, and then be accessed by the recipient, assuming they have the same software that the sender used to construct the attachments. This has great advantages over the unformatted stream of text which constitutes most email messages.

Two notes of caution:
- It is not advisable to send large files by email because it slows down

networks and many relay networks responsible for forwarding email may have size limitations, resulting in your email being rejected, or lost forever in the ether.

- Email is *not* secure. Thus the sending of sensitive medical data is not to be recommended unless precautions are taken to encrypt or make access to the data secure.

The lack of security associated with email makes it completely unsuitable for sending patient records, medical information on identified people or anything which you are not happy to have widely distributed. The process of sending

```
login: user02 (login to your local computer service)
Password:


Last login: Thu Apr 16 11:49:55 from liepad1


This machine holds your incoming electronic mail


Welcome to the Big University Computing Service
```
(automatically generated introductory message from your computer service)
```
% elm (typed by you to enter email program)
Mailbox is '/var/mail/user02' with 4 messages [ELM 2.4 PL23]
    1 Apr 14 BMJ              (256)   BMJ CONTENTS PAGE
O   2 Apr 14 R. Smith        (60)    message
O   3 Apr 14 B. Anderson     (55)    Hello
    4 Apr 10 BMJ              (301)   BMJ CONTENTS PAGE
```
(date delivered, sender)   (size)   (subject)
(list of your email messages)
```
|=pipe, !=shell, ?=help, <n>=set current to n, /=search pattern
a)lias, C)opy, c)hange folder, d)elete, e)dit, f)orward, g)roup
reply, m)ail, n)ext, o)ptions, p)rint, q)uit, r)eply, s)ave, t)ag,
u)ndelete, or e(x)it
```
(menu of email commands)
```

Command: Quit


% logout


CLI: Connection closed.
```

Figure 4.1 Typical remote user session. The entries in bold are those typed by the user

information electronically involves bouncing and copying it to various inter-mediary computer systems between the sender and recipient. The opportuni-ties for interception by a malicious third party are many and varied, and do not require enormous resources or intelligence. Without using a specific, recognised method of encryption before sending information electronically, and informing the recipient of the password to the encryption by means *other* than email, it is safer to trust the information to the conventional postal service, or 'snail-mail' in computer jargon.

The Worldwide Web (WWW)

The WWW is a recently developed method of interactively accessing infor-mation (web pages) via the Internet, on computers all over the world. It has advantages in that it has an attractive and easy to use interface and often incorporates graphics to enhance the information presented.

To use the WWW you will need a web browser, which is a program to allow you to access computers on the Internet and display the pages of infor-mation. There are several to choose from, and they are all regularly updated to include new features. Popular programs include Netscape, MS Explorer and Mosaic.

There are two modes of accessing the WWW. The big advantage of the WWW is the attractive graphical interface. Unfortunately, communicating such large graphics files between computers requires protocols normally only available on large computers (this method of rapid transfer is called transmis-sion control protocol/Internet protocol (TCP/IP)). To enable individual users to access these facilities there are two options:

- Running software on the remote computer, where your personal computer basically goes to sleep and just acts as a conduit for data communicated from your network provider's computer. That is, all the programs run on the remote computer and your personal computer acts as a screen to view the information.
- Software on your computer emulates the rapid connections present between larger computers, using protocols called serial line Internet protocol (SLIP) or point to point protocol (PPP). This means that the remote computer acts as a conduit for information/data being transferred between your computer and the Internet. All the programs run on your personal computer and the remote computer acts as a redirection point for the data coming from the Internet. This enables you to fully use your computer's capabilities, integrate your email and web programs and use your mouse for 'drag-and-drop' operations and so on. Such software is increasingly becoming an integral part of computers, for example, Microsoft Explorer and Microsoft Windows 98. This communication option requires your Internet provider to provide SLIP/PPP access and also requires a faster modem due to the large amounts of data being passed.

The Internet

Once set up and logged-on, you will be in your service provider's home page. A simple web page consists of a title and associated text and graphics. Embedded within the text are some words which are highlighted, usually by being in a different colour. These are links to other pages, which may be as close as the next page on the current site or refer to a page on the other side of the world. The power of the WWW is that its location makes no difference to the user. The question is no longer 'How do I get that relevant piece of information?' but 'Do I want access to it?'. If so, then it can be accessed instantly. By moving the mouse cursor over a link, the link text will then change colour and the address of the page to which it is pointing will appear on your web browser. When the mouse button is pressed, while over the link, your web browser will attempt to access that page by finding the website and downloading its contents. This will result in the piece of text identifying the link changing colour, to indicate you have accessed it. As navigation of web pages often involves clicking the 'back' button, when the page you get to may not be where you want to be, the colour change makes it obvious which links you have been to. Most web browsers will 'remember' the last few web pages you accessed. The colours of the text links may be defined by the site you are accessing or the set-up of your browser, depending on particular configurations. All being well, you will now be on a different site and you will have successfully 'surfed the net'. You can now access the links on the new page or go back to try other links.

Obviously, serendipitous random site hopping may result in some highly relevant and unexpected information being accessed, but the rapidly changing and expanding nature of the WWW requires a rational approach to information searching.

Searching for information on the WWW

As there is so much information on the Internet, organisations have set up websites with programs which allow you to search for information. These are called search engines and they regularly scour the Internet for information, gathering it into a database for easy searching. Searching is very easy; one simply types in a word and clicks on the search button. The major search engine sites are:

- Yahoo   http://www.yahoo.com/
- AltaVista   http://altavista.com/
- Excite   http://www.excite.com/
- Excite UK   http://www.excite.co.uk/
- HotBot   http://www.hotbot.com/
- Lycos   http://www.lycos.com/
- Infoseek   http://www.infoseek.co.uk/

No matter how obscure your subject, the biggest problem in searching the net will be selectivity, as most web searches result in thousands of hits. The various search engine sites offer different degrees of selectivity, such as by site (for example, only sites in the UK), or by date, or by language (as the net is not totally Anglocentric). There are various advantages and disadvantages to each of these sites and trying each one will determine the most useful one for you, such as the most refined search, or the fastest, or the largest numbers of responses or 'hits', depending on your particular subject and search strategy.

Medical resources

The above search engine sites are useful for general searches, but some sites provide a service to particular interest groups by gathering sites of relevance to, for example, biologists or medics. The amount of medical information available on the WWW is enormous, as is demonstrated by searching on almost any medical term. Some of the more relevant sites are listed in Table 4.1. As the web by its very nature changes quickly, these addresses are subject to change. The websites of grant-giving bodies are listed in Chapter 19.

FTP

FTP stands for 'file transfer protocol' and is a computer program used, as the name suggests, to transfer files between computers. Since computers and networks were invented, there has built up an enormous amount of freely accessible software and text files. These are files and programs which are not commercial products and which can be used without any direct payment. The software ranges from utility programs which perform simple tasks, to large and complex operating systems for expert users, together with an enormous amount of textual information on every possible subject. The software can be divided into two main types:

- **freeware**, which can be downloaded and used indefinitely, free of charge
- **shareware**, which must be paid for if used beyond an introductory period of 30 days or more than a few times. The fee tends to be modest, often less than US$50 (the currency of the net is usually US dollars or credit cards).

Most shareware programs are completely operational versions of software, many of which are as good, or better, than commercial programs which are much more expensive. Other programs are limited and can only be used for a limited period or a limited number of times, or certain functions such as saving or printing may be disabled. This is done as an incentive to pay your fees, whereupon a fully operational version will be sent to you. This is on par with the 'demo' versions of commercial software packages.

FTP allows you to retrieve these files to your own computer rapidly from sites which allow FTP access. Although FTP programs exist for smaller

Table 4.1   Websites of interest

Site	Site address
Centre for Evidence-based Medicine	http://cebm.jr2.ox.ac.uk/
Cambridge Public Health	http://fester.his.path.ac/uk/phealth/phweb.html/
York Centre for Health Economics	http://www.york.ac.uk/inst/che/
Centers for Disease Control (CDC)	http://www.cdc.gov/
The Cochrane Collaboration	http://hiru.mcmaster.ca/cochrane/default.htm
UK Health Technology Assessment Programme	http://www.soton.ac.uk/~wi/hta/
Centre for Reviews and Dissemination Databases	http://www.york.ac.uk/inst/crd/
National Library of Medicine (US)	http://www.nlm.nih.gov/
Food and Drug Administration (FDA)	http://www.fda.gov/
National Institute of Health (NIH – US)	http://www.nih.gov/
Royal College of Obstetricians and Gynaecologists	http://www.rcog.org.uk
World Health Organization (WHO)	http://www.who.ch/

Journals

British Medical Journal	http://www.bmj.com/bmj/
Lancet	http://www.thelancet.com/newlancet/
Health Economics	http://www.york.ac.uk/inst/che/he.htm
Pharmacoeconomics	http://topgun.adis.co.nz/11/.pe
Bandolier	http://www.jr2.ox.ac.uk/Bandolier/
Evidence-based Purchasing	http://www.epi.bris.ac.uk/publicat/ebpurch/index.htm

Other resources

The Global Health Network	http://info.pitt.edu/HOME/GHNet/
Health Web Medicine	http://www.ghsl.nwu.edu/healthweb/subj-med.html
Health Information Research Unit, McMaster University, Hamilton, Canada	http://hiru.mcmaster.ca/
Sudden Infant Death Syndrome (SIDS) Network	http://sids-network.org/index.htm
AIDS Information and Treatments	http://www.hopkins-aids.edu/
Public Health Resources	http://www.lib.umich.edu/hw/public.health.html
US Office of Disease Prevention and Health Promotion	http://odphp.oash.dhhs.gov/
US Association for Health Services Research	http://www.ahsr.org/
MED Guide (medical education)	http://kernighan.imc.akh-wien.ac.at/stz/plattner/txt/medgde.html
WAIS databases in medical science	http://www.ub2.lu.se/auto_new/auto_3.html

computers, the power of FTP lies in transfers between computers with high speed links, which are usually central Unix computers. To access a remote computer one normally needs to be a registered user, but to facilitate the free exchange of information and software, anonymous access is allowed to many FTP sites. This allows limited access to a remote computer using the user name 'anonymous', and typing your email address as your password, e.g. user2@computer.ac.uk. This access allows you to change directories, list the files stored on the FTP site and retrieve files from the site. As each remote FTP site uses different operating systems (normally some version of Unix) and different file conventions, you are advised to get the relevant information on the site first. This information will often be in the file called 'readme', or you will be directed to its location when you log-in. An example of an FTP session is given in Figure 4.2.

Most files archived on such services are compressed using one of a seemingly ever-increasing number of techniques. The last three letters of the file name sometimes give a clue as to the compression method in use:

- .gz, .shar and .tar are Unix compression methods
- .zip, .zoo, .arc and .lhz are all DOS or Windows compressed files
- .sit and .hqx are Mac compressed files.

Luckily the programs to decompress these files are widely available from FTP sites (in uncompressed form) or are distributed with computers. The main things to note about FTP are:

- Check your disk space on the computer account that you are transferring the file to, as Unix accounts are often assumed only to be used for email and so have limited file space. Also check the file you are getting to ensure it is not too big for you to handle; getting a 5MB file in a matter of seconds is wonderful, but not if the modem link between your Unix account and your personal computer takes hours to download the file.
- Remember the difference between binary and text files as they are handled differently by networks and FTP. Although some compressed files may be transferred as text files it is best to check local file conventions on the site you are transferring from, as incorrectly transferred files may be unusable.
- It is very unlikely that any of the files you download will have viruses on them, but it is essential to get some anti-virus software to check the files before using them.

Some anonymous FTP sites have local rules, so please obey them otherwise anonymous access will be removed. Some also have useful commands to automatically remove compression while downloading, or to search the site for an individual file, so it is always worthwhile looking for local information when logged in. Some useful sites are listed below:

- sunsite.doc.ic.ac.uk (a very large site which archives a lot of files)

```
login: user02  (login to your local computer service)
Password:
Last login: Thu Apr 16 11:49:55 from liepad1

This machine holds your incoming electronic mail

Welcome to the Big University Computing Service
(automatically generated login message)

% ftp
ftp> open big.ftp.site.ac.uk
Connected to big.ftp.site.ac.uk.
220 big.ftp.site.ac.uk FTP server (Version wu-2.4.2-academ[BETA-13](5)
Tue Jul 29 22:09:53 BST 1997) ready.
(login message from remote site)
Name (big.ftp.site.ac.uk:user02): anonymous
331 Guest login ok, send your complete email address as password.
Password: (here you type your email address, e.g. me@here.com)
230-Please read the file README for local info
230 Guest login ok, access restrictions apply. (successfully logged-in to
the site)
ftp> ls (lists the files available at the site)
200 PORT command successful.
150 Opening ASCII mode data connection for file list.
README
bin
biology
computing
science
unix
usenet
weather
pub
226 Transfer complete.
458 bytes received in 0.035 seconds (13 Kbytes/s)
(file listing of the directory you are in on the remote site)
ftp> get README (command to copy the file README to your local site)
200 PORT command successful.
150 Opening ASCII mode data connection for README (2015 bytes).
(starting transfer)
226 Transfer complete.
local: README remote: README

2098 bytes received in 0.022 seconds (91 Kbytes/s) (completing transfer)
ftp> bye (logging-out of remote site)
221 Goodbye.
% ls (listing files on your computer)
Mail/ README (retrieved file)
% logout (logging-out of your local site)

Connection closed.
```

Figure 4.2 An example FTP session. The entries in bold are those typed in by the user

- ftp.funet.fi
- micros.hensa.ac.uk
- ftp.winsite.com
- ftp.w3.org
- wuarchive.wustl.edu

Searching for files

As the number of sites and number of files grows inexorably, rational search methods have been invented. An excellent program for searching for files available by FTP is 'archie' which will perform a similar task to the WWW search engines described above, but centring on FTP sites. Figure 4.3 shows a sample session; searching for the file twsk21e.zip. Archie sites include:

- archie.doc.ic.ac.uk
- archie.hensa.ac.uk

In order to access a remote site running archie, the program 'telnet' is used. This is a program which can be run on Unix systems (versions are also available for PCs). It allows access to a remote computer but you must have a valid user name and password, if necessary, to log-in to a remote computer using this program. For most of the sites running archie, using the user name archie is enough. There is also a website for archie searches: http://archie.hensa.ac.uk/archie.html.

Usenet

Usenet is the debating theatre of the Internet. It consists of a number of themed discussion groups, or newsgroups, covering everything from archaeology to zoology. If you have something you want a lot of people to read, you can post it to a suitable newsgroup and wait for a response. The response can be as a reply to the newsgroup, or to you if you give your email address. Some groups are very active and you can expect replies in less than 24 hours from anywhere in the world. One of the more relevant groups is the sci.med newsgroup, which has an increasing number of participants on numerous specialist topics. There is a web resource listing the current medical newsgroups at http://www.shef.ac.uk/~nhcon or
http://www.geocities.com/HotSprings/1505/hrnewsgroups.html.
There are several broad categories of groups:

- bionet   biology
- biz   business
- comp   computers
- misc   miscellania
- news   usenet
- rec   hobbies and games
- sci   science

```
login: user02  (login to your local computer service)
Password:


% telnet archie.doc.ic.ac.uk  (command to connect to an 'archie' service)
Trying 193.63.255.1...
Connected to phoenix.doc.ic.ac.uk.
Escape character is '^]'.
                    SunSITE Northern Europe
   Located at the Department of Computing, Imperial College, London.
                (automatically generated login message)
.

.

.

    To access archie,    login as archie    no password
    To access the source area connect to sunsite.doc.ic.ac.uk

To abandon this login, enter a control-D
Note the erase character is DEL and erase line is control-U
It is now 6:06PM on Thursday, 16 April 1998
UNIX(r) System V Release 4.0 (phoenix.doc.ic.ac.uk)

login: archie  (your login)
# Bunyip Information Systems, Inc., 1993, 1994, 1995

# Terminal type set to `vt100 24 80'.
# `erase' character is `^?'.
# `search' (type string) has the value `sub'.
(successfully logged-in to archie service and list of the default parameters)
archie.doc.ic.ac.uk> prog twsk21e.zip  (command to search for 'twsk21e.zip')
# Search type: sub.
# Your queue position: 1
# Estimated time for completion: 5 seconds.
working... = (searching for your file)

Host ftp.imar.ro (193.226.4.129)
Last updated 05:02 25 Feb 1998

Location: /pub/trieste/win3.x/winsock-1/stacks/TrumpetWinSock
FILE -rw-r--r-- 305674 bytes 00:00 28 Feb 1997 twsk21e.zip

Host ftp.be.schule.de (192.76.176.140)
Last updated 05:48 31 Jan 1998

Location: /pub/windows
FILE -rw-r--r-- 1134541 bytes 22:00 22 Dec 1996 twsk21e.zip
.................[lots more hits deleted to save space] (results of your search)

archie.doc.ic.ac.uk> bye  (logging-out of archie service)
# Bye.
Connection closed by foreign host.
```

Figure 4.3 Sample searching session

- soc   social groups
- talk   politics.

There are also those starting with alt which tend to be sensitive or controversial areas, such as sex, extreme political views, drugs and other 'alternative' subjects. The usenet is an enormous source of information; there are FAQs or 'frequently asked questions' files which can be a source of very useful information to the new user. The details of how to read, post and download messages are beyond the scope of this brief introduction, but many guides are available throughout the Internet.

Conclusion

This is a short introduction to the capabilities of the Internet. The best way to investigate it is to try it out. A useful site to visit is http://lcweb.loc.gov/global/internet/training.html which contains a list of Internet guides and tutorials to get you started. A taste of what is possible using the Internet can be found in a recent paper (Johnson *et al.* 1998), which uses the WWW to transfer medical images for emergency clinical management worldwide. It is, of course, available on-line as well: http://www.bmj.com/cgi/content/full/316/7136/988.

Reference

Johnson, D.S., Rajinder, P.G., Birtwistle, P. and Hirst, P. (1998) Transferring medical images on the world wide web for emergency clinical management: a case report. *BMJ* **316**, 988–9

## 5

An introduction to effective literature searching and medical library resources

Patricia C. Want

Within the wider context of UK library and information services, librarians working in the health sector are generally acknowledged to have been among the first to see the potential of new technology. By the end of the 1970s, most had come to terms with the challenges and opportunities offered by widespread computerised access to medical information. In particular, the familiar bulky volumes of printed *Index Medicus*, formerly painstakingly hand-searched, began to make way for Medline database access, which required the mastery of new search skills. Thus, through working with medical literature on a daily basis, in some cases over several years, many librarians have become expert searchers and are prepared to offer help and guidance as required.

Numerous published guides to the effective use of resources have been produced by medical librarians over the past six decades; only recently has user demand become a key element in furthering the educational process. Reasons for this include widespread individual access to electronic databases hitherto only readily available via libraries and a growing emphasis on the effective use of information resources to establish evidence bases for clinical decision-making.

Much useful information still appears in printed form. The information seeker should be aware of the fact that many such resources, which include a number of statistical publications, remain for the time being the preferred option for speedy and successful resolution of certain inquiries.

The three resources most likely to be accessed by the novice searcher are:

- Medline
- the Internet
- *The Cochrane Library*.

This chapter describes basic search techniques which can be applied to the first two categories and provides a brief summary of the UK medical library network. Search techniques applicable to *The Cochrane Library* on CD-ROM are fully described in Chapter 6. Since the summer of 1998, *The Cochrane Library* has been accessible using a standard Internet browser but as the facility is available only on subscription the CD-ROM version is likely to remain the preferred option for libraries. The most recent quarterly release containing abstracts of Cochrane reviews is freely accessible at the following website:

(http://www.update-software.com/ccweb/cochrane/cdsr.htm).

Approaching an enquiry

Most librarians favour a structured approach in the first instance; this applies whether searching Medline, *The Cochrane Library* or some other database, or when browsing a library's online catalogue under author, keyword, subject heading or title for a particular book or serial publication. An understanding of how controlled (thesaurus) headings are applied for each resource is an advantage and might repay further investigation on the part of the novice searcher; free text should always be used with caution for subject searching, owing to the limitations of natural language, such as the prevalence of synonyms.

If results are unexpectedly poor, the exploration of possible alternative options may yield results. Whether or not they do so, the process of investigation is in itself part of the learning curve. Unearthing information frequently incorporates an element of serendipity; even the most experienced researcher from time to time discovers useful information only incidentally.

If assistance is required, a medical librarian may be able to identify hitherto unsuspected sources of information and, depending upon the depth of information needed, may suggest approaching external resources. At this point, the right of access may arise, since libraries having a different type of funding source may be unable to offer ready access to a non-contributor. For example, an individual employed exclusively on an NHS contract cannot necessarily assume free access to academic library facilities and vice versa. The cross-sectoral divide is not easily overcome but initiatives are under way to find mutually acceptable solutions. One collaborative venture involving a university library and several local NHS trusts is set to be implemented early in 1999. Meanwhile, it is advisable to make preliminary enquiries concerning available options and obtain beforehand any formal authorisation which may be applicable. Access to independently funded libraries is normally restricted to the appropriate fee-paying membership with the proviso that libraries containing important subject collections will normally provide access to suitably accredited researchers for a stated purpose, primarily for the purpose of historical research.

Proficiency in searching comes only with constant practice; regular users benefit from keeping up to speed with newly introduced search terms and database innovations. However, given time constraints within the medical profession it may be that, beyond a certain level, inter-professional co-operation is essential if worthwhile search results are to be achieved. Opinion conflicts as to whether the medically qualified end-user searches the literature as efficiently as librarians working in the health sector and a number of studies have examined this question (Wanke and Hewison 1988; McGibbon *et al.* 1990; Haynes *et al.* 1994). The former has the advantage of in-depth medical knowledge, the latter of formal training in the principles upon which information is indexed and organised for retrieval purposes and familiarity with the vagaries of database usage from working with such resources on a daily basis.

Searching Medline

Medicine as a discipline has benefited greatly from the rich bibliographic resources provided by the National Library of Medicine in the USA, originally the Library of the Surgeon General's Office, US Army. These run in continuity from the original Index Catalogue, first published in 1880, to Medline and associated current databases.

Medline is the preferred starting point for most individuals conducting their own literature searches. It may be accessed free of charge via the Internet, bearing in mind that basic telecommunication charges apply for the duration of the connection, or via a terminal in a medical library which subscribes to the service and provides the facility either locally networked or on a stand-alone PC with multiple CD-ROM drives. Commercial providers may also offer subscriber access via the Internet. The library of the British Medical Association, in conjunction with a commercial provider, offers Medline access to personal members. A comprehensive list of options is available on the OMNI website: (http://omni.uk/general-info/internet_medline. html).

PubMed (http://www.ncbi.nlm.nih.gov/PubMed), provided by the US National Library of Medicine (NLM), is generally considered to provide the best 'free' Medline service. Certainly, for currency of citations it is the preferred option since it incorporates PreMedline which comprises in-process citations not yet fully processed for inclusion in the full Medline database. A second interface option from NLM is Internet Grateful Med (http://igm.nlm. nih.gov/) offering free access not only to Medline but also to several other NLM databases. These include Popline, a database devoted to abortion, family planning and related topics, citations having been selected from a wider range of primary sources than the journals indexed on Medline. In March 1998, it was estimated that 7.6 million searches were carried out on the two NLM services, more than were identified during the whole of 1996 (7.4 million) (National Library of Medicine 1998). PubMed has recently been appraised in a short paper (Agnostelis 1998) concluding that, whereas PubMed offers an important means of searching from the desktop, local networked versions may well be preferred for more complex searches or those which entail searching large numbers of citations.

PubMed allows the use of the Boolean operators 'and', 'or' and 'not' to assist in refining searches and pull-down menus enable specific fields to be searched. Hypertext links to citations on related subjects and also to full-text journals are available, although the latter may not permit access to more than the abstract unless the journal concerned is part of a current subscription. A 'clinical query' filter option enables any of the following four categories to be applied:

- therapy
- diagnosis
- etiology (note the spelling – the system will not accept 'ae' in the subheading)
- prognosis.

With effect from the beginning of August 1998, the speed of the system has been dramatically enhanced. Further refinements will shortly be introduced, including new search filters. Additional 'limits' options in a redesigned Advanced Search page include 'English language', 'Human' and 'Age Groups'. The PubMed and Internet Grateful Med web pages, respectively, should be consulted from time to time for news of the latest planned refinements. The National Library of Medicine has arrangements with a number of publishers to provide full-text links to articles in over 300 periodical publications. A list of titles may be viewed at http://www.ncbi.nlm.nih.gov/PubMed/jbrowser.html. Conditions of use are dictated by the publishers themselves so non-subscribers may find they are unable to proceed further than the contents pages or abstracts of articles; occasionally the full text of an article is available free of charge or may be viewed for a fee. Papers published in the *BMJ* are now becoming freely available on the web. Thus, wherever an article in the *BMJ* is immediately accessible via PubMed a button labelled 'Free BMJ' now appears. Click on the button to read the paper concerned and follow through any relevant links offered in 'hypertext', that is, text which is underlined or otherwise highlighted, indicating that mouse-clicking the word will lead to related information.

Medline on CD-ROM provides the searcher with access to a more sophisticated search tool, of particular value for complex searches, with which as yet the free alternatives do not compete in terms of the full range of search options. It may incorporate features such as a facility permitting the participating library to alert the user to journals held in its collection. The difficulties encountered in accessing the Internet at peak periods are also avoided. CD-ROMs are normally updated monthly, so searches may need to be 'topped up' by scanning PreMedline. CD-ROM Medline providers include Ovid, the Dialog Corporation and SilverPlatter.

Perhaps the most important aid to searching Medline effectively is its controlled thesaurus of subject headings which are 'treed' in hierarchical fashion. It should be noted that the indexing system is highly sophisticated and that specific rather than general terms are allotted. To each citation a number of thesaurus headings are attached, some of which are defined as being the 'focus' or major point of the article. Papers on a single topic can be refined by the use of such 'focus' headings, usually designated with an asterisk. A number of designated 'fields' aid further refinement of a search. These include subheadings such as 'drug therapy', 'etiology', 'pathology' and 'surgery', among many others. A list of more advanced search options includes, for example, the facility to search gene symbols, molecular sequences and individual subheadings ('floating' subheadings). Where two or more concepts are to be linked in a compound search, the 'focus' and 'subheading' options should be allotted with caution, since over-zealous refinement may result in relevant citations being missed.

Various strategies have been devised for the identification of reviews and meta-analyses on Medline, such as those prepared by the University of York NHS Centre for Reviews and Dissemination, which can be used both on Medline and CINAHL (Cumulative Index to Nursing and Allied Health Literature). Details are available on its web page (http://www.york.ac.uk/inst/ crd/search.htm). Another useful source of guidance to research strategy options and methodological search filters is to be found on the web page for the Institute of Health Sciences Library, University of Oxford (http://www. ox.ac.uk/library/filters.html). These have been developed in two formats, for Ovid and Silverplatter, and can be downloaded.

Perhaps the greatest pitfall for the unwary is the injudicious use of text words. Despite helpful inbuilt links to subject headings (mapping), such links do not always function successfully. The novice searcher often overlooks the precision of the system and a disregard of synonyms and of changes of spelling between singular and plural are common errors. It may also be necessary to allow for differences between English and American spelling; using instead an appropriate subject heading ensures that relevant articles are retrieved in a single search statement. An expectation that acronyms alone are sufficient to recover all related information is also unfounded. For example, PET is just as likely to retrieve information on tabby cats in a veterinary journal as pre-eclamptic toxaemia in an obstetric publication.

To take a further example, hormone replacement therapy (HRT) is indexed on Medline with the MeSH (Medical Subject Heading) 'estrogen replacement therapy'. In August 1998 the results found in Table 5.1 were posted, using OVID search software, under a selection of terms which might be input by the random searcher. Of these, depending upon the nature of the original enquiry,

	Term	Results	Type of term
Table 5.1	**Results of a Medline search for 'HRT'**		
1	Estrogen replacement therapy	2287	MeSH Heading
2	*Estrogen replacement therapy	1653	MeSH Heading + 'focus' option
3	HRT	576	Text word
4	Hormone replacement therapy	1173	Text word
5	Estrogen replacement therapy	439	Text word
6	Oestrogen replacement therapy	55	Text word

Table 5.2 Subheadings posted for search statement: *estrogen replacement therapy	
Subheading	No. of references
Adverse effects	277
Contraindications	24
Economics	4
History	1
Instrumentation	1
Methods	125
Mortality	2
Nursing	2
Psychology	34
Standards	20
Statistics and numerical data	16
Trends	6
Utilisation	33

a skilled searcher familiar with the literature, anticipating a high number of postings, would probably commence a search by inputting automatically statement no. 2. A search of greater complexity, requiring the use of several search terms, may require the user to employ instead statement no. 1.

The subheadings in Table 5.2 were posted for search statement no. 2, but these should always be applied with caution when combining multiple search statements.

A search statement may be further refined to specify 'English language', 'Human' (to exclude experimental work on animals) and 'Review Articles', the latter currently defined for all NLM databases as 'all review types: Review literature; Review of Reported Cases; Review, Academic; Review, Multicase; and Review, Tutorial'. Many searchers, especially in the academic sector, will have ready access to a selection of electronically published journals via the local network. As with the more familiar printed versions, availability is entirely dependent upon a subscription having been purchased by the university or NHS library concerned, or perhaps personally by a regular user. Wherever a link with an electronic journal is readily available this should be evident and an active link will have been established enabling the Medline searcher to access full-text articles in place of the usual abstracts. A systems librarian or other member of the library staff familiar with local database provision will normally readily provide instruction to the novice searcher and indicate how to access those journals which are locally available online.

Searching the Internet

Internet access is readily available in most medical libraries. Once basic navigational skills have been acquired, these are best honed by constant practice.

The Internet serves both as a communication tool and as a means of transmitting and retrieving information. Clearly, it has potential value as an educational medium but the lack, at present, of any form of quality control on the mass of websites appearing daily limits its usefulness. Informed estimates reveal that some 20 million new pages are being added to the web each month, providing a clear indication of the scale of the problem. Potentially useful sites are easily overlooked in a mass of information overload and the process of distinguishing the useful from the superfluous can be burdensome. The user, while delighted at the prospect of direct access to important documents, can soon become discouraged at the inordinate length of time it takes to download bulky publications.

The pitfalls of natural language searching become apparent almost immediately and are, in fact, magnified on the Internet where, language barriers aside, literacy on the part of neither the searcher nor the information provider is a prerequisite. The author's attention was recently drawn to an instance where inadvertent input of a misspelled word revealed sites more useful than with the term spelled correctly. It is clearly unwise to assume that only keywords favoured by the user will achieve the desired results.

Search engines are programs set up on the Internet to aid navigation, but users should be aware that each covers only a percentage of available sites. Most can be used with ease and are relatively fast, but not all lend themselves to any kind of structured searching.

There is no 'best' search engine or web directory and, thus, familiarity with more than one is advisable. The leading contenders are identified with their addresses in Chapter 4. All have a US bias but the web directory Yahoo (www.yahoo.com) is a popular choice since it retrieves UK medical material reasonably well, as does the search engine AltaVista (altavista.digital.com). Sometimes, devices can be employed which help to pinpoint sites more accurately, such as the insertion of inverted commas surrounding compound terms. Meta-search engines allow simultaneous searching of several search engines at once, but limit flexibility and are probably best avoided by the beginner.

Of major concern to the medical library and information community is the indiscriminate provision of information on the Internet. In November 1995, OMNI (http://omni.ac.uk) was launched. OMNI is a gateway providing comprehensive coverage of UK medical sites and the best resources worldwide; all sites described meet stated evaluation criteria. By 19 August 1998, some 3548 resources had been included. Medical Matrix (http://www.medmatrix.org) offers access to further resources worldwide.

Internet discussion lists (mailing lists) provide a forum for communicating electronically with other subject specialists without charge. Lists may be open to any participant or 'closed' to a particular group. The Directory of Mailbase Lists Database (http://www.liszt.com) provides a guide to availability. Within the Uk, Mailbase list options can be viewed at http://www.mailbase.ac.uk.

The beginner is advised to develop a quick reference list of key resource sites by judicious use of 'Bookmarks' (Netscape) or 'Favorites' (Microsoft Explorer) so they may be speedily consulted at need. Sometimes only the most relevant section need be stored. Good housekeeping practice is advisable and the temptation to accumulate endless website addresses should be resisted. Favoured addresses are best organised and stored in named subject folders for quick reference. A lengthy miscellaneous list soon becomes unwieldy. Stored addresses should be reviewed from time to time and any which have altered or sites no longer of interest should be deleted.

Full-text documents are often published electronically in the form of compressed text or 'Portable Document Format', more frequently referred to by the acronym PDF. The microscopic print can only be read satisfactorily with a pdf viewer, commonly Adobe Acrobat, which can be readily installed free of charge and retained. It is available from the adobe website at http://www.adobe.com. A web browser can be configured to recognise pdf files so that the viewer automatically becomes operational whenever such files are encountered.

Medical library provision in the UK

Quality of services
A document entitled *Accreditation of library and information services in the health sector: a checklist to support assessment* has been developed by the Accreditation Working Group of the Health Panel of the Library and Information Co-operation Council (LINC Health Panel 1998). This checklist is intended for use across all sectors of health library provision in England and Wales, in order to encourage the adoption of agreed standards in respect of study facilities offered by individual libraries. The document includes, among endorsing bodies, the Conference of Postgraduate Medical Deans of the United Kingdom (COPMED) and the King's Fund.

Local and regional provision
Regional library units within the NHS co-ordinate local library activities and provide support and training; examples are the North Thames Regional Library Service and the Anglia and Oxford Region Health Care Libraries Unit. Local library networks such as LASER (London And South East Region), HLN (Health Libraries North) and EMRLN (East Midlands Regional Library Network) facilitate inter-library transactions within defined boundaries. Numerous other co-operative schemes exist with varying degrees of formality which may be defined by, for example, library type, subject coverage or user group.

National provision
The British Library Document Supply Centre (BLDSC) in Boston Spa is a key national resource for photocopies of articles and the loan of books and journal

issues to registered libraries. Holdings include conference proceedings, theses and report literature. Payment is by means of a system of prepaid forms and requests are normally sent by post or transmitted electronically via ARTTEL (Automated Request Transmission by Telecommunications). Resources can also be accessed internationally via the BLDSC if such intensive pursuit of a document is warranted, but it is costly.

Royal College and Society libraries

This important category embraces the libraries of the Royal Society of Medicine (RSM) the British Medical Association (BMA) and those Royal Colleges with significant collections. They are independently funded, so have an obligation to provide library services to the designated, fee-paying, membership, who contribute towards their upkeep. However, requests for discretionary access to special collections by suitably accredited researchers, particularly for the purpose of medico-historical research, are rarely denied, although terms and conditions may differ.

Between them, these libraries hold a rich and diverse range of both current and historical resources. All have arrangements in place, varying in formality, which enable them to be used as a discretionary resource as the need arises. They play an important part in supporting health library provision across the UK, in providing a significant back-up resource through the designated channels for those seeking references from the less common books and journals which might be highly specialised, non-current or published in languages other than English.

Conclusion

Medical library users, once introduced to the range of key printed and electronic resources available in their respective university, hospital library or postgraduate centre, should be suitably equipped to resolve straightforward enquiries with little further assistance. The onus is then upon the individual researcher to develop such skills to the extent most helpful to them in the course of their day-to-day commitments and medical librarians are happy to assist in this process. The adoption of a process of self-accreditation within NHS libraries would help to ensure standard minimum provision. Fellows and Members of Royal College libraries, many of whom are scattered throughout the UK or are overseas, may also rely upon the in-depth special subject knowledge of library staff to obtain more specialised information where required as an adjunct to local library provision.

References

Anagostelis, B. (1998) PubMed: free Medline from the National Library of Medicine. He@lth *Information on the Internet* **1**, 6–7

Haynes, R.B., Walker, C.J., McKibbon, K.A., Johnston, M.E. and Willan, A.R. (1994) Performance of 27 MEDLINE systems tested by searches on clinical questions. *Journal of the American Medical Informatics Association* **1**, 285–95

LINC Health Panel (1998) *Accreditation of Library and Information Services in the Health Sector: A Checklist to Support Assessment.* London: LINC Health Panel Accreditation Working Group

McKibbon, K.A., Haynes, R.B., Dilks, C.J.W. *et al.* (1990) How good are clinical MEDLINE searches? A comparative study of clinical end-user and librarian searches. *Comp Biomed Res* **23**, 583–93

National Library of Medicine (1998) Online usage statistics smashed. *NLM Newsline* **53**, 1–2

Wanke, L.A. and Hewison, N.S. (1988) Comparative usefulness of MEDLINE searches performed by a drug information pharmacist and by medical librarians. *American Journal of Hospital Pharmacy* **45**, 2507–10

6

Using *The Cochrane Library*

Lelia M.M. Duley

The Cochrane Library is currently the best single source of evidence about the effects of health care. An electronic publication, it is available as a CD-ROM or floppy disk to be loaded on a personal computer or network, or it can be accessed via the Internet. Easily accessible and very user-friendly, even for the computer illiterate, it presents the work of members of the Cochrane Collaboration and others interested in assembling high quality evidence on the effects of health care. In the UK, *The Cochrane Library* is available in all National Health Service hospital libraries. In some hospitals it has also been introduced on to local computer networks, which makes it more readily available in a variety of clinical situations.

The information in *The Cochrane Library* includes:
- Cochrane Reviews and Protocols
- summaries and references to reviews published in paper form
- a register of controlled trials
- a register of methodology references.

With a growing awareness of the need for a more evidence-based health service, *The Cochrane Library* is increasingly being used to assist clinical decision-making and health policy, but it is also a very powerful research tool. For example, it now has far more references to randomised trials than Medline or any other bibliographic database.

This chapter will focus primarily on research applications of *The Cochrane Library*. As a background, the rationale for systematic reviews will be outlined, followed by a brief explanation of the history and aims of the Cochrane Collaboration. The contents of *The Cochrane Library* will then be described, with some examples to illustrate how the main databases can be used.

Rationale for systematic reviews

Systematic review of research evidence is an essential scientific activity, for which the rationale is now well established (Mulrow 1994; Collins *et al.* 1997). With over two million articles published every year in over 20 000 biomedical journals, it is impossible for any individual to stay up-to-date with primary research, even within a very specialised area. Increasingly, therefore, it is necessary to rely on reviews of research findings. Systematic reviews are valuable not only in clinical settings, but also to researchers. Reviews can be used to identify, justify and refine hypotheses, for example, and they help to identify and avoid pitfalls of previous work, estimate sample sizes and delineate adverse effects.

Systematic reviews are an efficient scientific tool. Although compiling a review may be time-consuming, it is likely to be quicker and less costly than doing a new study. Equally important, the review may actually demonstrate that another trial is unnecessary. Reviews can also speed the implementation of effective interventions and the withdrawal of ineffective or harmful interventions (Antman *et al.* 1992). The generalisability and consistency of research findings can be established and explored within systematic reviews. When reviews include a synthesis of data from individual studies (meta-analyses) then statistical power and precision will both be increased.

The Cochrane Collaboration

The Cochrane Collaboration is named after Archie Cochrane, a Scottish epidemiologist who worked in Wales for most of his life. In 1972, Cochrane published a radical critique of the health and social services, *Effectiveness and Efficiency: Random Reflections on Health Services*, which was to have far-reaching effects. In this book, he highlighted the absence of an adequate knowledge base for much of the care provided and made a strong case for the evaluation of new and existing forms of care in controlled trials which use randomisation to generate unbiased comparison groups. When the effects of an intervention are very large, as they were for example in the 1940s when penicillin was first introduced for the treatment of infected war wounds, carefully controlled research is rarely required. Usually, however, the best that can be expected is a more moderate benefit. In this situation, guidance is needed from systematically assembled, reliable research evidence. Cochrane's proposal was that such evidence is essential to inform the choices made within the health services by policy makers, practitioners and patients. Some years later, Cochrane acknowledged that a major obstacle to this process was the lack of ready access to reliable evidence about the effects of health care. He laid out a challenge, which has now been taken up by the international collaboration named after him:

> 'It is surely a great criticism of our profession that we have not organ-
> ised a critical summary, by speciality or subspeciality, adapted periodi-
> cally, of all relevant randomised trials' (Cochrane 1979).

Cochrane then awarded the wooden spoon to obstetrics, as the medical specialty which had made the least effort to seek good evidence on which to base its practices. This challenge was taken up by Iain Chalmers and his colleagues, who spearheaded an international collaborative effort to prepare systematic reviews, using statistical synthesis (meta-analysis) when this was appropriate and possible, of all randomised controlled trials relevant to care during pregnancy and childbirth. By the late 1980s, this work had led to the publication of books, papers and an electronic journal, *The Oxford Database of Perinatal Trials* (Chalmers 1988). In 1989, Cochrane referred to this systematic review of controlled trials in pregnancy and childbirth as 'a real milestone in the history of randomised controlled trials and in the evaluation of care', and he withdrew the wooden spoon.

Having demonstrated that this approach was possible for one specialty, the challenge was to see whether it was possible to extend this work to all areas of health care. In 1992, the first Cochrane Centre was opened in Oxford, with support from the NHS Research and Development Programme, and the Cochrane Collaboration was launched internationally one year later. The Cochrane Collaboration is an informal network of individuals which welcomes the involvement of anyone interested in contributing to the work. The aim of the Collaboration is to help people to make well-informed decisions about health care by preparing, maintaining and promoting the accessibility of systematic reviews of the effects of health care interventions. It is based on eight key principals (Chalmers *et al.* 1997):

- collaboration
- building on the enthusiasm of individuals
- avoiding duplication
- minimising bias
- keeping up-to-date
- striving for relevance
- promoting access
- ensuring quality.

The principal outputs of the collaboration are Cochrane Reviews. The process for conducting a systematic review is outlined in Table 6.1. Preparation and maintenance of Cochrane Reviews are the responsibility of members of collaborative review groups, of which there are now over 40. Members of these multi-disciplinary groups share an interest in a particular health problem, or group of health problems, such as the treatment of schizophrenia, prevention and treatment of menstrual disorders, or how best to care for people with dementia. Each collaborative review group is responsible for assembling and maintaining a register of controlled trials relevant to the scope of the group. As for any piece of research, the first step in preparing a systematic review is to develop a protocol. These Cochrane Protocols are published in *The Cochrane Database of Systematic Reviews* and are later replaced by the completed Cochrane Review. There is a comments and criticisms system built into the software, but feedback can also be sent directly to the authors and/or editors, as full contact details are available.

To assist in the preparation of systematic reviews, the Collaboration has published a Handbook: *How to Conduct a Cochrane Systematic Review* (Mulrow and Oxman 1997). This can be viewed in a hypertext format within *The*

Table 6.1. How to do a systematic review	
Developing the protocol	**Doing the review**
• State the objectives of the review.	• Search for studies that seem to meet eligibility criteria.
• Outline eligibility criteria for studies to be included: – types of study design – types of participant – types of intervention – types of outcomes.	• Tabulate characteristics and assess methodological quality of each study. • Apply eligibility criteria and justify any exclusions.
• Describe search strategy to identify potentially eligible studies.	• Assemble the most complete data set feasible. • Analyse results, using statistical synthesis of data (meta-analysis) if appropriate and possible.
• Describe methods for the review.	• Perform sensitivity analyses and subgroup analyses, if appropriate and possible.

Cochrane Library and a hard copy can also be printed from the text files. In addition, the Collaboration has 16 methods working groups. These are tackling a wide variety of issues, including statistical methods, diagnostic tests and placebo effects. Details of the work of each methods working group are available in *The Cochrane Library*.

What is in *The Cochrane Library?*

The Cochrane Library is updated every three months. It contains four main databases, briefly described below, along with several other useful documents and sources of information. The four databases are:
- the Cochrane Database of Systematic Reviews (CDSR)
- the Database of Reviews of Effectiveness (DARE)
- the Cochrane Controlled Trials Register (CCTR)
- the Cochrane Review Methodology Database.

CDSR

CDSR includes the full text and data of the regularly updated Cochrane Reviews. These reviews are presented in two sections: complete reviews and protocols. The protocols are for reviews currently being prepared (all include an expected date of completion). In Disk Issue 3, 1998, there were 428 reviews and 397 protocols.

Protocols consist of the background; objectives; search strategy and methods of the reviews, sections that will also be published in the subsequent, complete review. Reviews also have tables describing:
- the methods, participants, interventions and outcomes within each included study

- reasons why any apparently relevant study was excluded
- graphs which summarise the analyses within the review
- text to describe and comment on the results and the reviewers' judgements about the implications for practice and research.

The software allows the user to select the statistics for conducting meta-analyses within the reviews. For dichotomous data, the range of options includes odds ratios (with a choice of three different methods) relative risk and risk difference. For continuous data, the options are weighted mean difference and standard mean difference. There is also a choice for the confidence intervals: 90%, 95% or 99%.

The CDSR has a comments and criticisms system which allows the user to comment on any aspect of the review. Reviewers respond to these comments and a summary of the original comment and the reviewer's reply are published within the updated reviews. The big advantage of electronic publication is that the review itself can be amended to correct errors, to take account of comments from users of the review and to add new data.

DARE

DARE is prepared by the National Health Service Centre for Reviews and Dissemination at the University of York. This database provides information on reviews of the effectiveness of heath care interventions and ways of organising health care, published on paper. It includes three main types of records:

- Structured abstracts, assessing and summarising previously published systematic reviews judged to be of good methodological quality. In Disk Issue 3 1998 there were 572 of these records.
- ACP Journal Club abstracts of reviews, produced by the American College of Physicians Journal Club up to 1995. In Disk Issue 3 1998 there were 38 of these records.
- Source records, references to other published systematic reviews. These records include citations for reviews which have been quality assessed by the Centre for Reviews and Dissemination but did not meet at least one of their criteria for methodological quality (295 records) and older reviews which have not been assessed (802 records).

DARE aims to identify the best quality (non-Cochrane) systematic reviews. It complements the Cochrane Database of Systematic Reviews by offering a selection of quality assessed reviews and includes reviews of randomised trials as well as other sorts of study designs. DARE records include a brief critical appraisal of the review, offering an assessment of its methodology, describing the results and conclusions and commenting on any implications for the NHS. The citations are identified from weekly searches of Current Contents Clinical Medicine, monthly searches of Medline and CINAHL, annual searches of PsycLIT, Amed, ERIC and Biosis, hand-searching of key major medical journals and scanning of grey literature sources, such as conference abstracts, theses and dissertations for higher degrees and lay journals.

CCTR

CCTR includes over 190 000 references to controlled trials that might be relevant for inclusion in Cochrane Reviews. These records have been identified primarily through searches of the major electronic bibliographic databases (such as Medline, Embase and CINAHL) and hand-searching of health care journals within the Cochrane Collaboration. The emphasis in maintaining CCTR has been to maximise sensitivity, which means that there may be duplicates and some records may not refer to randomised or quasi-randomised trials. Nevertheless, CCTR is the best single source of information on controlled trials.

Disk Issue 3 1998 also introduced two new sections under the heading CCTR:

- *Medical Editors' Trial Amnesty* To minimise the effects of biased reporting, systematic reviews need to be based on as high a proportion as possible of relevant studies. Because of the potentially important health care consequences of excluding relevant unreported trials many of the world's major medical journals, including the *BMJ, The Lancet* and *Annals of Internal Medicine*, have joined together in calling an amnesty for unpublished trials. The amnesty was launched on 19 September 1997. In Disk Issue 3 1998 there were contact details for 150 unpublished trials.
- *About the CCTR* This section describes the CCTR and lists search engines and search tags used for coding references which are useful in searching.

Cochrane Review Methodology Database

This bibliography is of use to those new to the science of reviewing as well as those who are already immersed in it. Nearly 800 references include published reports of empirical studies of methods used in reviews, as well as methodological studies that are directly relevant to doing a review, such as empirical studies of the association between research methods and bias in randomised controlled trials. Books, conference proceedings and special journal issues devoted to the topic of systematic reviews and meta-analysis are included, as are articles introducing systematic reviews and meta-analysis to a wide audience and those which address specific issues of relevance.

Many of the references include an abstract and all have methodological keywords which makes it very easy to search for all papers on similar topics. Examples of the keywords include:

- meta-analysis – general discussion
- meta-analysis – sensitivity analysis
- meta-analysis – dichotomous data
- meta-analysis – continuous data
- data collection – blinding and reproducibility.

Other useful information within *The Cochrane Library* includes:

- Information about the Cochrane Collaboration. This section gives information about the work and scope of each of the 46 collaborative review groups and the 16 methods working groups, as well as information about the Cochrane centres and other Cochrane entities;
- Other sources of information.
- The Internet: this section lists various sources of health care information available on the Internet, along with the relevant hypertext links. 'The Cochrane Collaboration on the Internet' includes http://www.update-software.com/ccweb/cochrane/htm. This website provides information about *The Cochrane Library*, such as training materials, examples and frequently asked questions.
- INAHTA technology assessments, author abstracts: these are references to reports prepared by members of the International Network of Agencies for Health Technology Assessment (INAHTA), many with structured abstracts prepared by the authors. In Disk Issue 3 1998 there were 374 of these records.

Other information in *The Cochrane Library* includes:

- the User's Guide, which gives full instructions on how to use the software
- the Cochrane Handbook, which is a guide to preparing and maintaining a Cochrane Review
- a glossary of terms used within the Library.

Some examples of the research uses of *The Cochrane Library*

The Cochrane Library is a rich source of information about the effects of health care and about the science of systematic reviewing (research synthesis).

Doing systematic reviews

The main steps in planning and conducting a systematic review are summarised in Table 6.1. There are many ways in which *The Cochrane Library* can be helpful to anyone doing a systematic review, regardless of whether or not they are working within the Cochrane Collaboration. For example:

- developing the protocol for a review
- identifying relevant studies in CCTR
- developing a search strategy
- identifying systematic reviews
- constructing the review
- doing systematic reviews of observational data and data from evaluations of screening and diagnostic tests.

Developing the protocol for a review

The Cochrane Handbook, *How to Conduct a Cochrane Systematic Review*, outlines the key issues in developing a protocol for a systematic review. Although primarily written to guide those undertaking systematic reviews of randomised trials within the Cochrane Collaboration, the handbook contains much that is relevant to all reviews, regardless of the kinds of study design eligible for inclusion.

Identifying relevant studies in CCTR

The most difficult step in the conduct of any systematic review is often the identification of all relevant studies that should be considered for inclusion. A tremendous amount of work has been done within the Cochrane Collaboration to identify trials and this is now available to everyone through CCTR.

The search function in *The Cochrane Library* applies to all the databases simultaneously. Having clicked on the search icon on the left of the screen, there is a choice of a simple or an advanced search. The advanced search should be used for a comprehensive search. Records in CCTR include the relevant Medline or Embase accession numbers, and MeSH keywords have also been included for many of the records. Full and up-to-date instructions on how to use the search facility are included in the User's Guide, which is in a Word file on each CD-ROM.

Many of the references in CCTR also include the journal abstract and some of the references to conference abstracts include the actual abstract. This means that it is often not necessary to get the full paper or the book of abstracts in order to decide whether a study is potentially eligible for inclusion.

Developing a search strategy

For those who wish to search other bibliographic databases for relevant references, there is a considerable amount of information that may be helpful in developing and conducting a search strategy. For example:

- The Cochrane Handbook has a section on locating and selecting studies, which includes examples of search strategies for Medline, EMBASE, Science Citation Index, LILACS (Latin American and Caribbean Health Sciences Literature), Biological Abstracts and PsycLIT.
- The Cochrane Review Methodology Database includes references to papers which describe the sensitivity and precision of a search strategy to identify references to randomised controlled trials within Medline (Dickersin *et al.* 1994), which discuss the importance of subject terms (Counsell and Fraser 1995) and which point out that bibliographic databases can have bugs, just like any other software (Adams *et al.* 1992).
- There is a description of how each collaborative review group has developed and maintained its own specialist register of relevant references. These descriptions often include the methodological and/or subject terms used for general bibliographic databases, such as Medline, EMBASE and CINHAL (Cumulative Index of Nursing and Allied Health Literature).

Identifying systematic reviews

When planning a review, it is important to identify other relevant reviews as these can be a source of additional studies potentially eligible for inclusion in the review. In addition, looking at other reviews will often help to refine the questions still needing to be addressed and to identify hypotheses to be tested in the new review. Searching *The Cochrane Library* will identify not only Cochrane Reviews and Protocols, but also any reviews referred to in DARE. As well as the citation, many of the records in DARE contain structured abstracts of the published review.

Constructing the review

The Cochrane Collaboration has developed a Review Management software (RevMan) which enables Cochrane reviewers to construct their reviews. All Cochrane Reviews are compiled within RevMan and *The Cochrane Library* has details of the website where this software is available, free of charge. It can be downloaded and used by anyone, but software support is only available to people contributing reviews to the Cochrane Collaboration. Advantages of this software are that:

- it includes tables for displaying characteristics of the studies
- it can be useful for managing references and multiple citations to studies
- it has the capacity to do meta-analysis and display the results graphically.

These are all useful functions, even for reviews that will eventually be published only as paper reports.

Doing systematic reviews of observational data and data from evaluations of screening and diagnostic tests

The basic principles of a systematic review apply to reviews of all types of study and so the Cochrane Handbook is a useful resource for those conducting all types of review. Also, the Cochrane Review Methodology Database includes references to articles which summarise some of the issues in conducting these other sorts of reviews (for example, Irwig *et al.* 1995) and gives information about the relevant Cochrane methods working group. This information includes an outline of the scope and topics covered by the group, a list of reports they have published and any references to related work. Examples of reviews of these kinds of studies can also be found on DARE. Finally, the RevMan software can be used for compiling these reviews. It includes a data table which is designed to display data for which meta-analysis is not appropriate.

Planning a randomised trial

A systematic review summarising current knowledge is an essential component in the preparation for any primary research, including randomised trials. When planning a randomised trial, it is important to demonstrate that an important question remains unanswered and, therefore, that a new trial is justified. Additional advantages are that the systematic review will help to:

- formulate the question to be addressed in the new study
- highlight important outcomes
- generate estimates of the necessary sample size
- by describing the strengths and weaknesses of previous studies, provide insights into how the design of any new study could be improved.

For anyone planning a trial, *The Cochrane Library* is a rich source of information. In an increasing number of areas, a few minutes' search will either yield a high quality up-to-date review or, if the review is out of date, extending the search will quickly identify the studies required to update it. The following is an example of a logical sequence of inquiry to make maximum use of the library:

1 Search for completed reviews, looking in CDSR and DARE. If there is already an up-to-date review, it does not need to be done again. If a review is available but is not up-to-date, the CCTR can be searched to identify any additional studies, and these added to the review.
2 If no review is available, search CDSR for a protocol. The reviewer responsible for the protocol could also be contacted for further information.
3 If there is no review and no protocol on either database, search any Internet sites that may be relevant, such as ScHARR-Lock's Guide to the Evidence and the IDEA Database of Evidence-based Topics.
4 If no review is identified, use the Cochrane Handbook as a guide to developing a protocol for the review.
5 Search CCTR for potentially eligible studies. This greatly simplifies the search strategy, which is probably the most important component of any systematic review and, before the advent of CCTR, was often the most time-consuming.

Having summarised the currently available evidence, you are now in a position to design a randomised trial.

How to subscribe to *The Cochrane Library*

The Cochrane Library is an essential resource for anyone interested in doing systematic reviews, planning randomised trials, or understanding the rapidly evolving science of systematic reviewing. For information on how to subscribe, contact Update Software Ltd, Summertown Pavilion, Middle Way, Oxford OX2 7LG, UK. Fax: +44 1865 516918. Email: help@update.co.uk.

Acknowledgements

Thanks to Clive Adams, Iain Chalmers, Ruth Frankish, Julie Glanville, Sonja Henderson, Ellen Hodnett and Jim Neilson for helpful comments on earlier drafts of this chapter. Special thanks to Mark Starr for masterminding such wonderful and user-friendly software.

References

Adams, C.E., Lefebvre, C. and Chalmers, I. (1992) Bugs discovered during SilverPlatter Medline searches for RCTs. *Lancet* **340**, 915–16

Antman, E.M., Lau, J., Kupelnick, B., Mosteller, F. and Chalmers, T.C. (1992) A comparison of results of meta-analyses of randomized control trials and recommendations of experts. *JAMA* **268**, 240–8

Chalmers, I. (1988) *The Oxford Database of Perinatal Trials.* Oxford: Oxford University Press

Chalmers, I., Sackett, D. and Silagy, C. (1997) 'The Cochrane Collaboration' in: A. Maynard and I. Chalmers (Eds) *Non-random Reflections on Health Services: On the 25th Anniversary of Archie Cochrane's Effectiveness and Efficiency,* pp. 231–49. London: BMJ Publishing Group

Cochrane, A.L. (1972, reprinted 1989 in association with the BMJ) *Effectiveness and Efficiency: Random Reflections on Health Services.* London: Nuffield Provincial Hospitals Trust

Cochrane, A.L. (1979) '1931–1971: a critical review, with particular reference to the medical profession' in: *Medicines for the Year 2000,* pp. 1–11. London: Office of Health Economics

Cochrane, A.L. (1989) 'Foreword' in: I. Chalmers, M. Enkin and M.J.N.C. Keirse (Eds) *Effective Care in Pregnancy and Childbirth.* Oxford: Oxford University Press

Collins, R., Peto, R., Gray, R. and Parish, S. (1997) 'Large-scale randomised evidence: trials and overviews' in: A. Maynard and I. Chalmers (Eds) *Non-random Reflections on Health Services: on the 25th Anniversary of Archie Cochrane's Effectiveness and Efficiency,* pp. 197–230. London: BMJ Publishing Group

Counsell, C. and Fraser, H. (1995) Identifying relevant studies for systematic reviews. *BMJ* **310**, 126

Dickersin, K., Scherer, E. and Lefebvre, C. (1994) Identification of relevant studies for systematic reviews. *BMJ* **309**, 1286–91

Irwig, L., Macaskill, P., Glasziou, P. and Fahey, M. (1995) Meta-analytic methods for diagnostic test accuracy. *J Clin Epidemiol* **48**, 119–30

Mulrow, C.D. (1994) Rationale for systematic reviews. *BMJ* **309**, 597–9

Mulrow, C.D. and Oxman, A. (1997) The Cochrane Collaboration Handbook. How to conduct a Cochrane Systematic Review. *The Cochrane Library.*

Appendix

Searching *The Cochrane Library*

You cannot choose which database to search in *The Cochrane Library*, searches are always run against all databases and the list of results is then shown against each database.

Simple searching

- Click on the search button on the button bar to view the search options (Figure 6.1). All text is searched (for example, titles, abstracts, authors names, citations, keywords). Titles are selected only if ALL search terms are found in the *text* of the record. Word order and case are ignored. Punctuation and numbers other than years are ignored. Words must be three characters or longer, and words of 16 characters or more are truncated.
- Type in the word/s you want to search on.
- Click on the search button or press enter, the index window will appear, displaying in red the number of hits (Figure 6.2).

Combining terms: narrowing down your search

Multiple terms can be entered in the simple search window. The order is not important. *The Cochrane Library* will retrieve documents containing *all* the words entered, which is equivalent to using Boolean "AND". The search below is equivalent to "BLOOD" AND "PRESSURE" AND "STROKE". The order of words is irrelevant as words will be matched in documents wherever they occur.

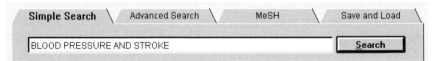

Words can be truncated by ending with "*" . For example, enter "ARTER*" and you will retrieve ARTERIAL, ARTERIES, etc. There is no left hand truncation.

The "NOT" operator can also be used to exclude records from your search.

Enter the word/s you want to search on here. All databases are searched and the results displayed in the index window with the numbers of hits in red.

Truncate using '*' (arter* will retrieve arterial, artery, etc.)

Enter several words, the order is not important. Searching is for documents containing all the words, anywhere in the document, not necessarily adjacent.

Use quotation marks to look for adjacent terms; compare searching for –ambulatory blood pressure – with "ambulatory blood pressure".

After entering your search, click the search button to start your search.

Click on these tabs to switch between search options.

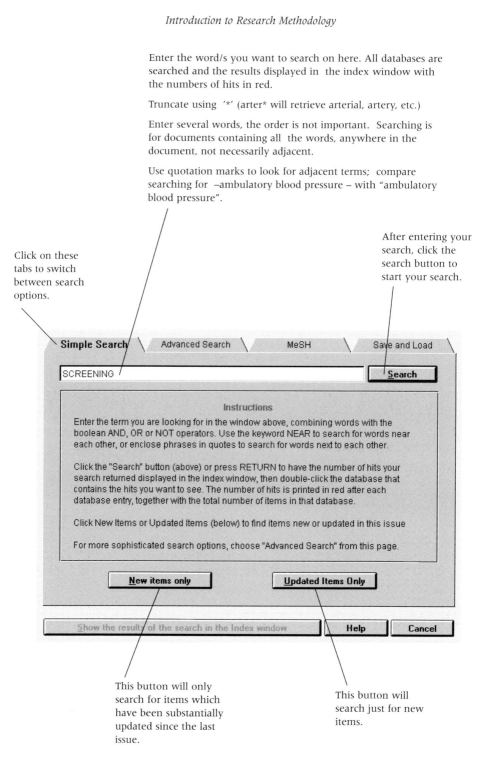

This button will only search for items which have been substantially updated since the last issue.

This button will search just for new items.

Figure 6.1 The 'Simple Search' screen

Numbers of hits for each database and total number of records.

Double click on the database headings to show individual documents. Double click again to collapse the view.

Double click on the document titles to display in the document window.

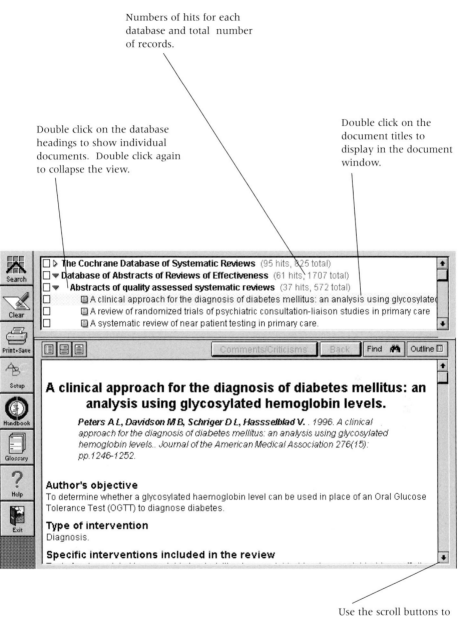

Use the scroll buttons to move down the document. To move between documents click on the titles in the index window.

Figure 6.2 Search results in the index window

Simple Search	Advanced Search	MeSH	Save and Load

"BREAST CANCER" NOT MALE	**Search**

Combining terms: broadening your search

You can use the Boolean operator "OR" in your searches to broaden out your search. This is useful if more than one word can be used for the same thing.

Simple Search	Advanced Search	MeSH	Save and Load

CANCER* OR NEOPLASM* OR ONCOLOGY	**Search**

Phrases and word proximity

Another way to narrow a search is to combine several words in a phrase, such as AMBULATORY BLOOD PRESSURE or MYOCARDIAL INFARCTION. Do this by placing the words used inside double quotes in the search box. This will give a different result to searching without the quotes because it will be interpreted as "AMBULATORY next to BLOOD next to PRESSURE" and will retrieve documents containing that complete phrase.

Simple Search	Advanced Search	MeSH	Save and Load

"AMBULATORY BLOOD PRESSURE"	**Search**

Alternatively, restrict searching by using the *near* operator, which acts like *and* but with the added condition that the entered terms must appear within six words of one another. For example, entering *stroke near units* will result in records being retrieved where *units* occurs within six words of *stroke*.

Simple Search	Advanced Search	MeSH	Save and Load

STROKE NEAR UNITS	**Search**

Advanced searching

The advanced search option allows complex queries to be built up step by step, with the results of each search being stored and then combined with other sets. It also gives access to additional features (Figure 6.3).

Combining several terms with "AND" and "OR"

'Advanced Search' allows more complex searches to be built up in stages, the results of each stage being saved in a numbered set (Figures 6.4 and 6.5). The

Click to display the
advanced search options.

Separate searches can be entered
and the results are stored as
numbered 'sets'. The number of hits
across all databases for each set is
shown in red.

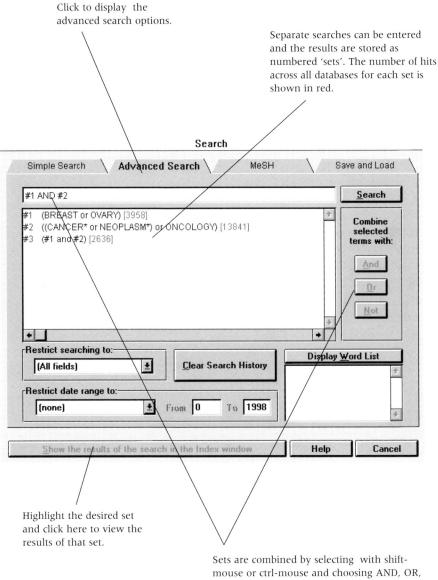

Search

| Simple Search | **Advanced Search** | MeSH | Save and Load |

#1 AND #2   **Search**

#1 (BREAST or OVARY) [3958]   **Combine**
#2 ((CANCER* or NEOPLASM*) or ONCOLOGY) [13841]   **selected**
#3 (#1 and #2) [2636]   **terms with:**

                                                       And

                                                       Or

                                                       Not

┌Restrict searching to:─┐   **Display Word List**
│ (All fields)   ▾│ **Clear Search History**
└───────────────────────┘
┌Restrict date range to:─┐
│ (none)   ▾│ From 0   To 1998
└────────────────────────┘

Show the results of the search in the Index window   **Help**   **Cancel**

Highlight the desired set
and click here to view the
results of that set.

Sets are combined by selecting with shift-
mouse or ctrl-mouse and choosing AND, OR,
NOT. Alternatively set numbers can be
entered manually in the search box.

Figure 6.3 The 'Advanced Search' screen

search shown in Figure 6.3 is equivalent to "(BREAST OR OVARY) AND
(CANCER OR ONCOLOGY OR NEOPLASM)"

● To save searches on the hard disk, click on 'Save and Load'.

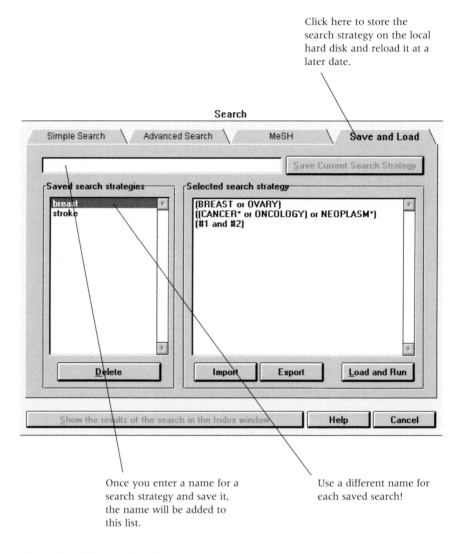

Click here to store the
search strategy on the local
hard disk and reload it at a
later date.

Once you enter a name for a
search strategy and save it,
the name will be added to
this list.

Use a different name for
each saved search!

Figure 6.4 'Save and Load' screen

MeSH searching

Keywords drawn from the MeSH Thesaurus published by the US National
Library of Medicine have been attached to many, but not all, records in *The
Cochrane Library*. For this reason, it is necessary to do a text search, as well as
a MeSH search, to carry out a complete interrogation of *The Cochrane Library*.
The MeSH Thesaurus is organised hierarchically in 'trees', with the lower
levels of the trees containing more specific terms. The MeSH search option
allows searching using the MeSH terms and tree structures.

The word list allows you to enter a
single term in the search box and view
index entries using that 'stem'. This
may help suggest alternative terms.

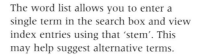

Search

| Simple Search | Advanced Search | MeSH | Save and Load |

STEROID   [Search]

#1   STEROID [1794]   Combine
                                                             selected
                                                             terms with:

                                                              [And]

                                                              [Or]

                                                              [Not]

Restrict searching to: [Clear Search History]   [Display Word List]
[(All fields)   ▼]   STEROID
                                                           STEROID-11-B
Restrict date range to: STEROID-17-A
[(none)   ▼]   From [0]   To [1998]   STEROID-21-M
                                                           STEROID-ABSE

Show the results of the search in the Index window   [Help]   [Cancel]

Searches can be restricted
to a particular field, or a
specific date range.

Figure 6.5   Other features of the advanced search screen

Step 1: Using the Permuted Index

The Permuted Index is an index of all the words that appear in the MeSH
thesaurus. It is used to locate specific MeSH headings:

- Open the MeSH search screen by clicking on the MeSH tab at the top of
  the screen.
- Open the Permuted Index by entering one word and clicking Thesaurus.
  All MeSH headings containing the word will then be displayed, in alpha-
  betical order.
- Locate the specific MeSH term you are interested in. Some terms are

followed by 'see' cross-references. Double-click on these terms to jump to the cross-referenced section of the Permuted Index.

- Double-click on a MeSH term to display the MeSH tree/s containing that term.

Step 2: Traversing MeSH trees

The MeSH trees containing the selected MeSH headings are displayed once a heading has been selected from the Permuted Index. These allow expanding or narrowing of the scope of the search, by selection of broader or narrower terms (Figure 6.6).

- To move up to a more general level in a MeSH tree, double-click on a term higher in the tree. Higher level terms are shown in bold (Figure 6.7).
- The more specific terms are displayed immediately underneath, and just to the right of your selected term. When other terms have more specific terms, this is represented by a number in parenthesis after the term, e.g. (+ 3). The number indicates how many headings appear lower in the tree. If there is no number, the term can not be expanded.

Step 3: Search

The final step is to search the database using the MeSH term selected. A MeSH term may appear in several MeSH trees. Esophageal Cyst, for example, occurs in both the Esophageal Diseases tree and the Neoplasms tree. There are therefore three search buttons:

- Click on 'Search This Term' to search on the exact term.
- Click on 'Search & Explode This Tree' to retrieve records indexed with the selected term plus any other terms appearing lower in the particular MeSH tree from which the term was selected.
- Click on 'Search & Explode All Trees' to retrieve the records indexed with the entered term plus all records indexed with terms appearing lower than the entered term in all MeSH trees containing that term.

The search will then be added to the search strategy with :ME after it, to indicate a MeSH term.

Note, some terms in the index are labelled '(Non MeSH)'. These terms are used by indexers to group headings in the MeSH tree structures and are not index terms *per se*. As they are not used to code individual records, Non-MeSH terms should only be used with the 'Explode This Tree' and 'Explode All Trees' search options.

Searching using field descriptors

Field descriptors are the code given to each field within a record, such as AU for author field, TI for title. It is possible to search using these field descriptors if you already know the MeSH term.

The permuted search window
lets you enter a single term.
It then returns all the terms
containing that term.

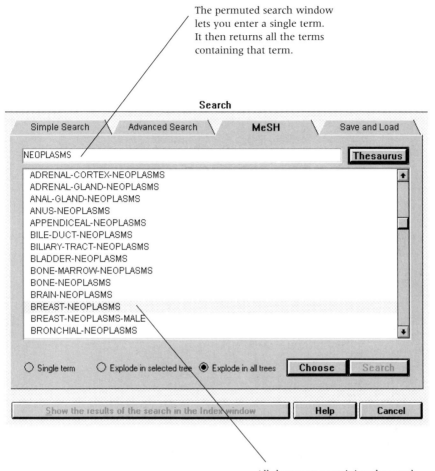

All the terms containing the word
'neoplasms' are listed alphabetically.
Double clicking on one of the terms,
or selecting it and clicking on the
choose button below, will take you
to the MeSH tree displays.

Figure 6.6 The MeSH search screen

Broadest terms are shown in bold.
Click on these to move up a level in
the MeSH hierarchy.

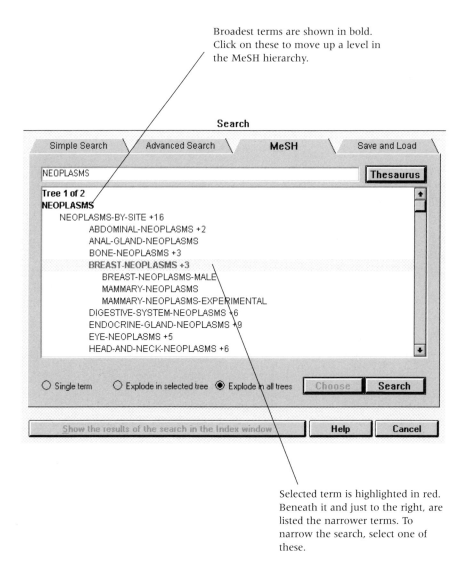

Selected term is highlighted in red.
Beneath it and just to the right, are
listed the narrower terms. To
narrow the search, select one of
these.

Figure 6.7 MeSH tree display

7

Critical appraisal of the research literature

Trish Greenhalgh

Research is the process of finding reliable answers to simple questions. Most biomedical research concerns quantitative studies (perhaps best exemplified by the randomised controlled trial) in which things are measured, counted and numerically compared with a view to confirming or refuting a specific hypothesis. In recent years, there has been increasing interest in the use of qualitative research, which adopts the techniques of the social sciences to gain an in-depth but non-numerical understanding of a particular topic and, perhaps, generate hypotheses that can then be tested in a quantitative study. Qualitative research is important but is beyond the scope of this brief chapter; its definition, application and limitations have been covered elsewhere (Mays and Pope 1996; Greenhalgh and Taylor 1997).

Critical appraisal is the process of looking at research findings with a view to answering three questions:

- Is this research valid (to what extent can I trust it)?
- Is it relevant (can I generalise the findings to my own practice)?
- What is the 'clinical bottom line' (should I change my practice and, if so, how)?

The research literature

Research evidence relevant to practising doctors usually falls into the category of either primary or secondary research evidence.

Primary

Primary (original and first-hand) research evidence comprises:

- *Randomised controlled trials:* most commonly, those which compare the effect of a drug treatment with that of placebo or a competitor.
- *Cohort studies:* in which subjects who have been exposed to a drug or toxin, such as a vaccine, tobacco or an environmental chemical, are followed up to see how many develop a particular disease or other outcome, compared with an unexposed cohort.
- *Case–control studies:* in which subjects who have developed a disease, as well as control subjects who have not, are asked about their exposure in the past to a putative causative agent.
- *Case reports:* in which a story about a particular event is told (most commonly these days, an adverse reaction to a drug).

- *Surveys:* in which something is measured in a group of patients (for instance, their blood pressure) or a group of health professionals (such as their knowledge or attitudes).

Secondary

Secondary research evidence, which is of particular interest to the busy clinician, is material that sets out to summarise and draw conclusions from primary studies; for example:

- *Journalistic (non-systematic) reviews:* which collect together some (but usually not all) primary evidence on a topic, usually interlaced with the author's personal opinion. Until recently, most overviews were written by experts in the field and presented in this format, which has been described as the tradition of 'eminence [*sic*] based health care'.
- *Systematic reviews:* in which all the evidence pertaining to a particular field of research has been collected via a systematic search of the literature and unpublished sources, and evaluated using predefined quality criteria.
- *Meta-analyses:* which are systematic reviews in which the numerical results of different studies have been combined using standard statistical techniques; for example, the recently published meta-analysis of the association between obstetric complications and the subsequent development of schizophrenia (Geddes and Lawrie 1995). Meta-analysis, simply by increasing the numbers in the calculations, can make the estimate of the effect of an intervention both more precise (the possible limits of its magnitude are more tightly defined) and more definitive (we can be much more confident that the result, whether positive or negative, is a true reflection of the effect studied rather than due to the play of chance).
- *Guidelines:* which have been defined as systematically developed statements to assist practitioner decisions about appropriate health care for specific clinical circumstances.
- *Economic analyses:* which are studies involving the use of mathematical techniques to define choices in resource allocation.

A piece of secondary research is only as good as the primary studies which went into it and the techniques used for making sense of those studies, so the notion that anything that bears the title 'systematic review' or 'meta-analysis' necessarily counts as high quality evidence is erroneous. Similarly, most clinicians are all too aware that guidelines issued with the best intentions may or may not be valid or practicable. Current published guidelines for most conditions are based more on expert consensus than on primary research evidence.

Asking answerable questions

A preliminary step towards 'appraising the evidence' on a topic is to formulate a simple, answerable question before you start pulling articles out of the medical literature. The clinical epidemiologists have exhorted us to redraft our clinical problems in the same language that researchers use to formulate their research hypotheses – that is, in terms of a three-part question (Sackett *et al.* 1991; Table 7.1). Clinical reality, of course, rarely lends itself naturally to such clean and simple formulations. For example, a woman contemplating the options for the place of birth for her first baby probably incorporates around 100 different factors into her final decision, including:

- evidence about survival statistics and caesarean section rates
- values (her own and other people's) such as an overall attitude to 'natural' or conventional medicine
- anecdotal experiences related by other new mothers at antenatal classes
- even the presence or absence of an accessible car park at the hospital.

There is currently much debate in academic circles about whether it is useful to deconstruct personal health decisions into their component facts and values, or whether we should accept that the paradigm of clinical epidemiology (the stuff of randomised controlled trials and their implications for individual patient decisions) can only address the simplest of issues and that the complexities of the lived experience of health and illness require a totally separate paradigm. Some authors (notably those whose specialty is decision science) argue that all health-related questions, no matter how complex, can be reduced to a series of dichotomous decisions, each of which can be addressed by a three-part question (Dowie 1996).

Others, myself included, believe that the toolkit of clinical epidemiology, while invaluable for providing precise answers to oversimplified questions such as that in Table 7.1, ceases to be useful when applied to a complex real-life question such as 'where should *we* have *our* baby?'. The latter question should, in my view, be addressed by the couple themselves using an inter-

Table 7.1 The three-part question	
Question	**Example**
1. How would I describe a group of patients similar to this one?	'In primiparous women aged between 20 and 30 and with no adverse family or personal medical history ...'
2a. What intervention am I considering?	'... would planned home delivery ...'
2b. What comparison intervention am I considering?	'... compared with planned delivery by a midwife in a consultant-led obstetric unit ...'
3. What are the most important and relevant outcomes?	'... lead to significant differences in maternal or fetal survival, neonatal morbidity, bonding and parental satisfaction with the birth?'

pretative paradigm, by discussing the options and integrating their personal values and preferences with research-based evidence through dialogue and reflection (Greenhalgh and Hurwitz 1998).

Whichever one of these theoretical standpoints you share, evidence has an important role to play. You will thus need to start with either a three-part question or some other structured and focused formulation and prioritisation of the clinical problems arising from the case. This is the step that is most often omitted in so-called evidence-based practice, resulting in what Grimley-Evans (1995) has termed 'evidence *biased* medicine' (the foolish and naïve attempt to address one clinical question by means of research evidence that pertains to a different question).

Decide what sort of research evidence you need to address your question

Most clinical questions that arise from individual doctor–patient (or health professional–patient) encounters tend to be about interventions, particularly diagnostic tests (including the clinical examination itself as well as technical investigations) and treatments (including drug therapy, surgery, counselling, and so on). Other important questions about individual patients include those about prognosis (what is likely to happen to a patient with condition X?). Questions arising from a public health or economic perspective may include practical issues of service delivery and the relative costs of different policies or protocols when applied to populations.

In general, questions about diagnostic tests should be answered by recourse to research studies that compare the test in question with a 'gold standard' in a defined, representative population. For example, the value of the triple test in prenatal screening for Down syndrome can be determined by offering the test to a sample of pregnant women and undertaking chromosomal analysis on the fetal tissue – either at amniocentesis or after birth (Cuckle 1996). The karyotype gives (or excludes) the diagnosis of Down syndrome with near 100% accuracy and the results of this test can be compared with those of the triple test to provide figures for:

- sensitivity (the extent to which the new test correctly picks up those with the condition)
- specificity (the extent to which it correctly excludes those without the condition)
- positive predictive value (if the test is positive, what the chance is that the patient actually has the condition).

These aspects of diagnostic test validation are discussed further elsewhere (Sackett *et al.* 1991; Greenhalgh 1997).

If the clinical question concerns a therapeutic (or preventative) intervention, the appropriate research design is virtually always a randomised controlled trial, or meta-analysis of randomised trials, for reasons that have been well rehearsed elsewhere (Bero and Rennie 1996) and are discussed later in this chapter.

Questions about prognosis are best answered not by randomised controlled trials but by a long-term (longitudinal) follow-up of a carefully assembled inception cohort. An appropriate cohort would be a group of individuals who share a particular feature (for example, a report of CIN I on a routine cervical smear) who are then followed-up to see what proportion recovers, stays the same or goes on to develop definitive disease. The prognosis of a condition as determined by a longitudinal cohort study will be heavily influenced by the sampling procedure. For example, a group of women in whom CIN I is detected in sexually transmitted disease clinics may well have a different prognosis from women diagnosed with the same condition in general practice, mainly because of the presence of confounding variables (see below). Hence, you should pay particular attention to the first part of your three-part question, 'How would I describe a group of patients similar to this one?', when seeking prognostic evidence from cohort studies.

Many 'public health'-type questions (that is, those which address the design and delivery of health care for a population rather than in an individual clinical decision) are also addressed through either randomised controlled trials or cohort studies. However, there is fierce debate about the ability of these methods to provide useful and practical answers to questions about community-based health promotion and/or models of service delivery. These complex issues, some authors argue, are better analysed using a qualitative or 'developmental' theoretical framework, in which lessons can be learnt about the process of change as well as about final outcomes. These issues are not considered further here but the interested reader is invited to pursue the relevant references (Speller *et al.* 1997; Britton *et al.* 1998; Greenhalgh 1998).

Searching the literature

Having formulated your question, the next step is to make sure that you have the best evidence in front of you. A counsel of perfection would be to undertake a systematic literature search on your chosen topic, including the growing range of electronic medical databases, a hand search of the specialist journals, a search for recently published articles in the *Science Citation Index* and personal correspondence with leading researchers in the field (Chalmers and Altman 1995) and with the pharmaceutical industry for negative unpublished papers. In practice, this process would take days or weeks and an acceptable compromise is to perform, with the help of a medical librarian if necessary, a search of the Medline, Cochrane (Bero and Rennie 1995) and perhaps 'Best Evidence' databases (Hunt and McKibbon 1997) using carefully selected subject headings and text words. This step should take between two and 15 minutes and will leave you with a manageable selection of articles to choose from.

Evaluating the methods section of published research: four pitfalls for the unwary

Table 7.2 shows a general checklist for evaluating the methods section of a research paper. A careful check through this list should detect the four main pitfalls in methodology: bias, confounding, power and validity.

Bias

Bias describes the systematic differences between groups that distort the comparisons between those groups. Bias is most obviously present in non-randomised trials in which comparison groups are allocated for convenience rather than at random – for example, all patients under consultant A receive one drug while those under consultant B receive a different drug. If consultant A's general approach to care differs from that of consultant B in important ways, differences in outcome would be wrongly attributed to differences in the efficacy of the drugs. Bias may also occur in randomised controlled trials if randomisation is not truly random or if the allocation to group is not concealed and if those assessing outcome are aware of which group the patient was in. The problems of bias in randomised trials are discussed further by Bero and Rennie (1996).

Table 7.2 Checklist for weighing up the 'methods' section of a published paper

1   Was the study original?

2   Whom is the study about?
  - How were subjects recruited?
  - Who was included in and who was excluded from the study?
  - Were the subjects studied in 'real life' circumstances?

3   Was the design of the study sensible?
  - What intervention or other manoeuvre was being considered?
  - What outcome(s) were measured and how?

4   Was the study adequately controlled?
  - If a 'randomised trial', was randomisation truly random?
  - If a cohort, case–control or other non-randomised comparative study, were the controls appropriate?
  - Were the groups comparable in all important aspects except for the variable being studied?
  - Was assessment of outcome (or, in a case–control study, allocation of case-ness) 'blind'?

5   Was the study large enough and continued for long enough and was follow-up complete enough, to make the results credible?

Reproduced with permission from Greenhalgh (1997)

Confounding

Confounding is where a measured effect attributed to a particular variable is in fact due to an unmeasured co-variable. For example, as mentioned earlier in this chapter, patients recruited from a sexually transmitted diseases clinic may be more likely to have one or more current sexual partners than those recruited from a GP's smear clinic. Subsequent differences between the groups in outcome after treatment for CIN I may be due to a difference in the interventions offered but may also be due to differences in sexual behaviour.

Power

Power is the ability of a study to detect a clinically significant difference between groups if one exists. A trial should be big enough to have a high chance of detecting as statistically significant a worthwhile effect, if it exists, and thus to be reasonably sure that no benefit exists if it is not found in the trial. There is no need to memorise the formula for calculating the power of a study, which is described in most basic textbooks on statistics (Altman 1991) and summarised in a recent *BMJ* (Campbell *et al.* 1995). It is important, however, to be aware of the three factors that influence the required sample size in a study: the nature of the primary outcome variable, the distribution of that variable in the study population and the size of a clinically significant change in that variable (what level of difference would you as a clinician deem important?).

For example, you might identify as a clinical problem the fact that a high proportion of infants born to Punjabi mothers who come to see you are underweight at birth and that many of these mothers are anaemic. In a randomised trial to measure the effect of iron supplementation, the outcome measure would clearly be the infants' birth weights, but how many patients should you randomise? The answer will depend on how much variation there is in the birth weight of newborn Punjabi infants without any prophylactic intervention, a factor generally expressed as the standard deviation of the variable. You would also have to decide what is an important (clinically significant) improvement in weight. Would a 2200 g infant have a substantially better chance than one of 1900 g, 2100 g or 2150 g? There is no mathematical formula for determining what is clinically significant, which is why a *statistically* significant result may or may not be clinically relevant.

Validity

Validity describes the overall ability of the methods used to answer the research question. This aspect is often best addressed using a combination of specific clinical knowledge and common sense. Do the methods appear clinically sensible? Have the authors failed to take into account factors that you would have expected them to look at? Have they used appropriate equipment and drugs? If you were looking at this research question would you have done it this way? Whereas the aspects described above are often decided by a statistician or an expert in evidence-based health care, overall validity is generally best assessed by an experienced clinician who is familiar with the particular problem being studied.

Evaluating the results: defining the strength of evidence

The defining characteristic of 'evidence-based' therapeutic decision-making as compared with traditional clinical methods is the use of mathematical estimates of probability and risk established from the average effect of the intervention in large population samples. It is beyond the scope of this chapter to discuss detailed statistical techniques for estimating such probability and risk, but clinicians should note some basic principles.

Until fairly recently, it was acceptable to look for the 'P values' in the results tables and count anything with $P < 0.05$ (less than 1 chance in 20 that this result occurred by chance) as a 'real' result. These days, P values are treated with increasing scepticism, especially when the number of comparisons performed by the authors exceeds about a dozen (making it quite likely that the result did arise by chance). It is generally felt that the results of research studies should not simply be classed as 'significant' or 'non-significant' but in terms of the likely magnitude of the effect of the intervention (point estimate of effect size) and the precision of this estimate.

The confidence interval around the effect size is, in effect, an estimate of the spread of results that might be found if the same experiment was repeated many hundreds of times. If the sample size was large, the actual result is very likely to reflect the true effect size. Conversely, small samples are more likely to produce extreme results through the play of chance. Hence, the larger the study, the narrower the confidence interval. If the confidence interval overlaps zero effect, either there is no real difference between the groups or the study is under-powered – that is, a larger study (or a meta-analysis) needs to be done. A clinically significant difference between the groups and a confidence interval that does not overlap zero effect suggests that the study is both positive (there is probably a real effect) and definitive (there is no need to repeat it).

Results of intervention trials are increasingly expressed in terms of numbers needed to treat (NNTs). The calculation of NNTs and other commonly used summary terms for the results of clinical trials is shown in Table 7.3 and discussed in more detail in specialist texts (Sackett *et al.* 1997; see also Chapter 15).

Conclusion

Critical appraisal skills are frequently equated with an 'evidence-based' approach to care. But evidence-based practice is much more than the ability to pick holes in published research papers. It is, many would argue, a way of thinking – an approach to systematically defining and addressing your own information needs and using that information appropriately and consistently in patient care.

Table 7.3 Illustration of mathematical estimate of benefit expressed as number needed to treat

The figures below are taken from a randomised controlled trial which compared the effect of aspirin plus heparin vs. aspirin in women with recurrent miscarriage and phospholipid antibodies (Rai et al. 1997). The equations are explained in more detail in Sackett et al. 1997.

	Miscarriage or stillbirth		Total
	Yes	No	
Control group (aspirin alone)	a = 26	b = 19	a + b = 45
Experimental group (aspirin plus heparin)	c = 13	d = 32	c + d = 45

Control event rate (CER)	= risk of outcome event (miscarriage or still birth) in control group = $a/(a + b)$; = 26/45; = 58%.
Experimental event rate (EER)	= risk of outcome event in experimental group = $c/(c + d)$; = 13/45; = 29%.
Absolute risk reduction (ARR)	= CER − EER; = 58 − 29; = 29%.
Relative risk reduction (RRR)	= (CER − EER)/CER; = 58 − 29/58; = 50%.
Number needed to treat (NNT)	= 1/ARR; = 1/(CER − EER); = 1/.29; = 3.4.

This shows that between three and four women need to receive heparin plus aspirin in order for one more live birth to occur, compared with the outcome on aspirin alone.

Many practitioners would argue that the really difficult part of evidence-based practice is to do with implementation, either at the level of the individual consultation, 'Did I remember to consider appropriate contraceptive advice for 15-year-old Ms Jones after her termination of pregnancy and, if so, what were the attitudinal, ethical and practical influences on the application of so-called best evidence?'; or at the level of departmental policy, 'Having looked up the evidence to make a decision about Ms Jones, what general policy should we adopt in this department for responding to a request by an under-age teenage smoker "to go on the Pill"?'.

The detailed analysis of how to implement change in professional practice and how to influence policy making for clinical effectiveness is beyond the scope of this chapter but this important subject is covered elsewhere (Appleby *et al.* 1995; Oxman *et al.* 1995; Dunning *et al.* 1998).

References

Altman, D. (1991) *Practical Statistics for Medical Research.* London: Chapman and Hall (the nomogram for calculating sample size or power is on page 456)

Appleby, J., Walshe, K. and Ham, C. (1995) *Acting on the Evidence: A Review of Clinical Effectiveness: Sources of Information, Dissemination and Implementation.* Birmingham: NAHAT

Bero, L.A. and Rennie, D. (1996) Influences on the quality of published drug studies. *International Journal of Health Technology Assessment* **12**, 209–37

Bero, L. and Rennie, D. (1995) The Cochrane Collaboration: preparing, maintaining, and disseminating systematic reviews of the effects of health care. *JAMA* **274**, 1935–8

Britton, A., Thorogood, M., Coombes, Y. and Lewando-Hundt, G. (1998) Search for evidence of effective health promotion. Quantitative outcome evaluation with qualitative process evaluation is best. *BMJ* **316**, 703

Campbell, M.J., Julious, S.A. and Altman, D.G. (1995) Estimating sample sizes for binary, ordered categorical, and continuous outcomes in two group comparisons. *BMJ* **311**, 1145–8

Chalmers, I. and Altman, D.G. (1995) *Systematic Reviews.* London: BMJ Publishing Group

Cuckle, H. (1996) Established markers in second trimester maternal serum. *Early Hum Dev* **47**, Suppl, S27–9

Dowie, J. (1996) 'Evidence-based', 'cost-effective' and 'preference-driven' medicine: decision analysis based medical decision making is the pre-requisite. *Journal of Health Service Research and Policy* **1**, 104–13

Dunning, M., Abi-Aad, G., Gilbert, D., Gillam, S. and Livett, H. (1998) *Turning Evidence into Everyday Practice: An Interim Report from the PACE Programme, November 1997.* London: King's Fund

Field, M.J. and Lohr, K.N. (1990) *Clinical Practice Guidelines: Direction of a New Agency.* Washington DC: Institute of Medicine

Geddes, J. and Lawrie, S.M. (1995) Obstetric complications and schizophrenia: a meta-analysis. *Br J Psychiatry* **167**, 786–93

Greenhalgh, T. (1997) 'Papers that report diagnostic or screening tests' in: T. Greenhalgh (Ed.) *How to Read a Paper: The Basics of Evidence-based Medicine*, pp. 97–110. London: BMJ Publishing Group

Greenhalgh, T. (1997) 'Searching the literature' in: T. Greenhalgh (Ed.) *How to Read a Paper: The Basics of Evidence-based Medicine*, pp. 14–33. London: BMJ Publishing Group

Greenhalgh, T. (1998) Meta-analysis is a blunt and potentially misleading instrument for analysing models of service delivery. *BMJ* **317**, 395–6

Greenhalgh, T. and Taylor, R. (1997) 'Papers that go beyond numbers' in T. Greenhalgh (Ed.) *How to Read a Paper: The Basics of Evidence-based Medicine*, pp. 151–62. London: BMJ Publishing Group

Greenhalgh, T. and Hurwitz, B. (1998) *Narrative Based Medicine: Dialogue and Discourse in Clinical Practice*. London: BMJ Publishing Group

Grimley Evans, J. (1995) Evidence-based and evidence-biased medicine. *Age Ageing* **24**, 461–3

Hunt, D.L. and McKibbon, K.A. (1997) Locating and appraising systematic reviews. *Ann Intern Med* **126**, 532–8

Mays, N. and Pope, C. (Eds) (1996) *Qualitative Research in Health Care*. London: BMJ Publishing Group

Oxman, A., Davis, D., Haynes, R.B. and Thomson, M.A. (1995) No magic bullets: a systematic review of 102 trials of interventions to help health professionals deliver services more effectively or efficiently. *CMAJ (Ottawa)* **153**, 1423–43

Rai, R., Cohen, H., Dave, M. and Regan, L. (1997) Randomised controlled trial of aspirin and aspirin plus heparin in pregnant women with recurrent miscarriage with phospholipid antibodies (or antiphospholipid antibodies). *BMJ* **314**, 253–7

Sackett, D.L., Haynes, R.B., Guyatt, G.H. and Tugwell, P. (1991) *Clinical Epidemiology – A Basic Science for Clinical Medicine*, 2nd edn. London: Little, Brown

Sackett, D.L., Richardson, W.S., Rosenberg, W. and Haynes, R.B. (1996) *Evidence-based Medicine: How to Practice and Teach EBM*. London: Churchill Livingstone

Speller, V., Learmonth, A. and Harrison, D. (1997) The search for evidence of effective health promotion. *BMJ* **315**, 361–3

## 8

Evidence-based medicine and getting research into practice

Cindy M. Farquhar

Evidence-based medicine (EBM) has become the catch-cry phrase of the 1990s. It is a popular focus for special workshops, conferences, textbooks, medical education and now frequently extends beyond clinical practice into purchasing and planning. This is best illustrated by the dramatic increase in medical literature on this topic. In 1997 and 1998 nearly 600 articles were indexed on Medline under the subject heading 'Evidence-based medicine', whereas prior to 1997 less than 300 articles in total had been published. The explosion of interest in this topic has occurred across a diverse range of specialties and backgrounds including medical, dental, nursing, educational and purchasing personnel.

It is a sign of EBM's growing impact on health-care practices that it has also attracted significant criticisms. There are concerns that it is merely serving health rationing. Some fear that it may interfere with individual clinicians' decisions by imposing rigid protocols. Others have argued that funding for research should not be directed to health services research and away from basic sciences. Yet others have suggested that it is a reductionist approach with no real concern for valid patient outcomes.

The other common sentiment, expressed by doctors and patients alike, is that surely doctors were always evidence-based? What were they taught at medical school if it was not based on evidence from research? Unfortunately, many surveys of differing practices have illustrated otherwise. The most familiar example of this was the failure of obstetricians to prescribe antenatal corticosteroids to women in preterm labour (Lewis *et al.* 1980; Keirse 1984), ignoring a growing body of evidence from randomised controlled trials (RCTs) which demonstrated clinical effectiveness (Crowley *et al.* 1990). In the area of gynaecology, surveys of prescribing patterns for heavy menstrual bleeding by both GPs (Coulter *et al.* 1995) and specialists (Farquhar and Kimble 1996) have shown either a lack of scientific knowledge of the topic or a complete disregard for the evidence. Evidence analysed thus far suggests that tranexamic acid is the most effective oral therapy while norethisterone is the least effective oral therapy, yet family doctors in the UK prescribe tranexamic acid in only 5% and norethisterone in 38% of cases (Coulter *et al.* 1995). Similar results have been reported from gynaecologists in New Zealand (Farquhar and Kimble 1996).

Definitions

EBM has been defined as 'the conscientious, explicit and judicious use of current best evidence in making decisions about the care of individual patients' (Sackett *et al.* 1996). It is about taking the best clinical evidence from systematic searching of the research evidence and translating it into individual expertise. To put it more simply, it is for those, medically trained or not, who want to put the results of scientific research into everyday health care.

For some clinicians, this has been interpreted as simply reading 'papers' and following the conclusions. However, this approach, which may have been satisfactory 30 years ago when medical literature and research was less prolific, is likely to fail because of the expansion of medical and scientific literature over recent years. For example, if you (a clinician) wished to find out the most effective medical treatment for heavy menstrual bleeding you may read a review article written by an 'expert' recommending norethisterone. Within this article you notice a lack of RCT data. You remember one RCT on the use of non-steroidal anti-inflammatory agents which demonstrated effectiveness. But basing management on one RCT may be misleading – the quality of the trial needs to be assessed: was the allocation of treatment concealed; how did they assess improvement? – and the type of patients included needs to be considered: how did they define heavy menstrual bleeding? Therefore, you decide to go a step further and look at other RCTs of medical treatment of heavy menstrual bleeding. You search Medline and find over 40 RCTs on the topic. How do you cope with this volume of research? Should all the papers be requested? Once the papers arrive how will their results be sifted and compared? It is an overwhelming task for any individual clinician to undertake in a short time frame. An alternative approach, which has now become popular (almost essential), is to seek reviews of the evidence that have been systematically prepared by a group of independent individuals and peer reviewed. Many such reviews of clinical therapeutics are now being published and in particular these are the main focus of the Cochrane Collaboration (see Chapter 6).

The essentials of EBM have been defined by Sackett and Haynes (1995). They include:

- asking the right questions
- finding the best level of evidence available
- appraising the evidence for quality and relevance
- implementing the results of the appraisal
- evaluating the changes in practice.

Formulating the question

Almost every time a clinician sees a patient, new information will be needed about some element of their care. Some of the questions are obvious (What is the diagnosis?) and some are easy to answer from reference books (What is the dose?). However, many times the questions will not be self-evident and time needs to be spent formulating the right question in order to track down the answers:

- Does this patient have risk factors?
- What is the prognosis for this condition?
- Which treatment is most effective in this particular patient?
- Which dosage is the most effective?
- Will this treatment cause more harm than benefit?

These questions are the starting point for using research evidence in everyday practice. Sackett *et al.* (1996) have described the elements of clinical questions:

- Define which patients the question is about.
- Define which intervention and, if necessary, an alternative intervention.
- Define which outcomes are of interest.

For example, your patient is a 40-year-old woman with heavy menstrual bleeding wanting advice about medical or surgical approaches.

Which patients?	Pre-menopausal women with regular heavy menstrual bleeding.
Which intervention?	Medical therapy.
An alternative intervention?	Endometrial ablation.
Which outcomes are desirable?	Reduction in heavy menstrual bleeding by pictorial bleeding assessment charts.

Finding the best level of evidence

Finding the evidence is the next step. Fortunately, this has been made easier by electronic searching. It is worth mentioning that there are many electronic databases. Search strategies have been developed to use them efficiently which are a science in themselves (Dickersin *et al.* 1995). Other sources of evidence include *The Cochrane Library*, which publishes a database solely of RCTs (mostly of interventions). It is the result of collaborative hand-searching efforts and electronic searching from many of the different review groups and centres of the Cochrane Collaboration. This may be a good place to start, especially if therapeutics is the question about which you are interested.

Appraising the evidence

In order for evidence to be reliable, a certain quality is required. The research methodology depends on what the research question is (Table 8.1). For example, the question of which is the most accurate diagnostic test for determining submucous fibroids in women is best answered by a comparative study of consecutive women with abnormal menstrual bleeding. A 'gold standard test' is compared with the new 'experimental test'; in this case, hysteroscopy is the gold standard and transvaginal ultrasound is the new test. Ideally, the new 'experimental test' should be conducted by an independent observer from the 'gold standard test' and the two observers should be

Table 8.1 The research question and the preferred research methodology	
Diagnostics (Is this new test valid and reliable?)	Cross-sectional surveys of new test and gold standard test
Screening (Should we use this as a screening test?)	Cross-sectional survey at pre-symptomatic stage of patients at risk
Prognostics (What is the long-term outcome of this particular diagnosis?)	Longitudinal cohort study of patients who have been diagnosed with early stage of disease
Causative (What are the risk factors for this condition?)	Cohort or case–control study
Therapy (How effective or harmful is this therapy?)	Randomised controlled trial

unaware of each others' results. The data should be collected in a prospective manner. In the area of prognostics, the best research design includes repeated observations of individuals with an early stage condition over a reasonable time frame (longitudinal cohort study). For example, in order to study natural history of endometrial hyperplasia, repeated endometrial samples should be taken over a limited time in the absence of intervention. Studies of natural history can be difficult to conduct because of the concern about untreated disease; careful scrutiny by an ethics committee is essential, as is informed consent of all patients taking part. Clear guidelines for withdrawal from the study when abnormalities are deteted is essential (see Chapter 17 for more on ethics committees).

In the area of therapeutic interventions, RCTs are considered to be the most powerful research design available to determine effectiveness (Sackett *et al.* 1991). Studies in which treatment is not allocated by randomisation tend to report larger treatment effects compared with randomised trials, often with higher numbers of false positives (Sacks *et al.* 1983). Not all interventions and treatments require RCTs. Sometimes, when the effects of care are dramatic, such research is unnecessary. For example, management of a woman with a severe prolapse will usually require a surgical procedure; similarly, the woman who is repeatedly severely anaemic in association with heavy menstrual bleeding will probably benefit from a hysterectomy and a woman with an ovarian mass which is at risk of torsion or other complications is recommended to undergo surgical removal of the mass. However, where there is doubt about the best approach, for example in the use of antifibrinolytic agents, then RCTs are necessary to determine the most effective therapy. When more than one RCT is available, then a systematic review should be sought (see Chapter 6). In some instances, the differences between health-care interventions may be the cost or side effect profiles and these also need to be systematically evaluated. For example, in the management of endometriosis there is little discernible difference between the different forms of medical suppression on the outcomes of painful symptoms. However, there are notable differences when side effect profiles are taken into consideration.

The Cochrane Collaboration is focused on identifying reliable evidence and preparing systematic reviews of therapeutic interventions using randomised controlled trials (see Chapter 6). Collaborative review groups have evolved, which cover most areas of health care. There are currently over 40 Cochrane Review Groups around the globe and the seven of them which deal directly with the field of obstetrics and gynaecology are:

- Cochrane Pregnancy and Childbirth Group
- Cochrane Menstrual Disorders and Subfertility Group
- Cochrane Incontinence Group
- Cochrane Gynaecological Cancer Group
- Cochrane Fertility Regulation Group
- Cochrane Neonatal Group
- Cochrane Breast Cancer Group.

Nearly 200 systematic reviews relevant to the specialty of obstetrics and gynaecology are currently available in *The Cochrane Library* and a similar number are at protocol stage. A systematic review is one in which a systematic approach has been applied to identifying all the relevant RCTs, asking a research question, extracting the data and creating a systematic report, which is published both electronically and often in scientific publications. This is available as both a CD-ROM and on the Internet. It is probably the best source of evidence currently available because the process attempts to reduce all possible forms of bias.

After assessing the quality of evidence, the clinician needs to consider the relevance of the evidence. In many cases, research has been focused on outcomes that may be of interest to the researcher, but are of no value in clinical decision-making. There are many examples of this in obstetrics and gynaecology. For example, there are over 20 RCTs of women on hormone replacement therapy where the outcome of interest is lipid profiles. Yet the real outcome of interest is morbidity or mortality from cardiovascular disease. An abnormal lipid profile does not necessarily equate with clinical disease. Other examples are:

- the use of barriers as a prevention strategy for adhesion formation in subfertility surgery, yet failing to report pregnancy data
- the studies of menstrual blood loss reduction with medical management of heavy menstrual bleeding which frequently ignore patient satisfaction.

The many studies reporting bone mineral density indices without reporting fracture rates are further examples. Another criticism is that studies often fail to provide evidence of other important effects of treatment. For example, outcomes such as venous thrombosis, breast cancer and endometrial cancer were not reported in the early studies of hormone replacement therapy, yet these outcomes may profoundly affect the quality of life, both during and after treatment.

In many instances, there will be no reliable or relevant research evidence available to guide decisions about health care. Ideally, in these circumstances, properly controlled research should be undertaken and patients entered into these trials. As this is not always possible, the next level of evidence should be used in clinical decision-making.

The NHS has accepted levels of evidence as follows:
- based on randomised controls
- based on other robust experimental or observational studies
- based on more limited evidence, but the advice relies on expert opinion and has the endorsement of respected authorities (Mann 1996).

In therapeutics, this depends on large cohorts which are often compared to a selected control group. It is important to note that the control group and the study group are likely to differ in their presenting symptoms or demographics in some aspect. Finally, if no reliable case series or cohort studies are available, then the decision is based on expert opinion or consensus opinion. In reality, our decision-making is frequently not even based on expert opinion or consensus but more on anecdotes and case histories that have become imprinted on our clinical memories. Clinicians concerned with providing the best level of care will reject decision-making on this basis. As the process of EBM becomes enmeshed in our way of thinking and more research (both primary and secondary) is undertaken, it is hoped that clinical decision-making will be less dependent on this level of evidence.

How to implement research findings

Gathering and publishing reliable evidence does not ensure that patients are always offered optimal care. Numerous discrepancies exist between what is considered to be the most effective care and what occurs in reality. There have been various attempts to address these issues in different ways. One of these is the 'Getting Research into Practice and Purchasing' project (GRiPP), which has developed critical appraisal workshops to help purchasers in the UK make use of reliable research. Other local groups have developed, but perhaps the most obvious movement has been the development of clinical guidelines.

Clinical practice guidelines have been defined as 'systematically defined statements to assist practitioner and patient decisions about appropriate health care for specific clinical circumstances' (Field and Lohr 1990). They represent an attempt to assess a large body of medical knowledge in a convenient, readily useable format. Like systematic reviews, they gather, appraise and combine evidence. However, most go beyond a systematic review in attempting to address all the questions relevant to clinical decision-making for a particular topic. Guidelines differ from decision analyses by relying more on reasoning and should offer a certain amount of flexibility. The real advantage of evidence-based clinical guidelines is that they should incorporate evidence from many different sources of research – diagnostics, prognostics and therapeutics.

Guidelines have also come in for a good deal of criticism. The following comments have been made of them:

- They restrict clinical practice and reduce it to a series of decision points.
- They only provide a middle level of practice instead of best practice.
- They are inflexible and unable to accommodate local conditions.
- They are political acts by managers keen to introduce cost saving.

One of the most commonly asked questions is 'Have guidelines resulted in better clinical practice?' Fortunately this question has been answered by a systematic review of RCTs and 'other robust designs' which demonstrated improvements in care and better patient outcomes (Grimshaw and Russell 1993). All but four of 59 published evaluations of clinical guidelines reported significant improvements in care and patient outcomes. Determinants of successful guidelines were also assessed and the development strategy, the dissemination strategy and the implementation strategy all influenced final patient outcomes. Guidelines that had been developed by those who were going to use them, that were linked to specific educational packages and that had patient specific prompts at the time of consultation, had a greater likelihood of succeeding (Grimshaw and Russell 1993).

Clinical guidelines should also undergo critical appraisal. The following questions should be asked of clinical guidelines:

- Were conflicts of interest addressed?
- Are they topic-based guidelines with objectives related to health?
- Was a multi-disciplinary approach taken which included an expert in EBM?
- Did identification and sifting of all relevant data occur and are the conclusions in keeping with the data?
- Do the guidelines deal with variations in medical practice?
- Are the guidelines valid and reliable?
- Are the guidelines clinically relevant, comprehensive and flexible?
- Do the guidelines take cost into consideration?
- Do the guidelines consider implementation strategies and review?

Ideally, guidelines are developed by individuals who represent multi-disciplinary groups, who agree independently to review all the available evidence from research and produce a simple format for the use of practitioners and patients alike. They should be peer-reviewed and tested and the evidence in each guideline should be accompanied by a grading of the levels of evidence. A useful clinical guideline should be based on scientific evidence from well-designed research which has been systematically assessed. The value of alternative practices should allow health practitioners, in a reasonably short amount of time, to make links between multiple options and outcomes. It is hoped that, with consistent reporting of guidelines development, systematic methods will prevail, making the guidelines more accessible and useful for their users. Finally, guideline evaluation should emphasise the need for audit of specific outcomes after a specifed time period.

Barriers to implementation

The following barriers to incorporating guidelines into everyday practice have been identified. There may be:

- genuine disagreement about the quality of the evidence
- an inability to accept the concept of levels of evidence
- an over-riding concern about medico-legal issues (over-ordering and over-treatment)
- personal preferences
- economic constraints and financial uncertainties
- failure of guidelines to be easy to use
- failure of patients to accept changes in practice
- a lack of patient-specific feedback (Greenhalgh 1997).

One author concluded that the successful introduction of guidelines needs 'careful attention to the principles of change management: in particular, leadership, energy, avoidance of unnecessary uncertainty, good communication, and, above all, time' (Ayers et al. 1995).

How to change clinical practice

Examples of the failure of the health profession to take heed of evidence from RCTs and well-designed studies have already been discussed earlier in this chapter. The topic of changing the behaviour of health professionals is the focus of a Cochrane Group (recently renamed the Effective Practice and Organisation of Care). A systematic review of how to change health professionals' behaviour has concluded that 'there are no "magic bullets" for improving the quality of health care, but there is a wide range of interventions available that, if used appropriately, could lead to important improvements in professional practice and patient outcomes' (Oxman et al. 1995). The interventions that were shown to be most effective included the use of outreach visits and local opinion leaders. Dissemination-only strategies, such as conferences or the mailing of unsolicited materials, were the least effective approaches.

Implementation strategies by health care organisations have also been analysed. As most groups now have a structure for quality improvements, mechanisms can be developed to monitor progress in this area. Many of these initiatives are relatively new and assessment of their success is ongoing. The GRiPP initiative of the Anglia and Oxford Regional Health Authority in the UK has a number of projects under assessment, including the use of dilatation and curettage in women with heavy periods and the use of corticosteroids in preterm labour (Dunning *et al.* 1994; Appleby *et al.* 1995).

An evaluation of the GRiPP project noted the following points:

- Prerequisites for implementing changes in clinical practice are nationally available research evidence and clear, robust and local justification for change.
- There should be consultation and involvement of all interested parties, led by a respected product champion.
- The knock-on effect of change in one sector (for example, acute services) on others (such as general practice or community care) should be examined.
- Information about current practice and the effect of change needs to be available.
- Relationships between purchasers and providers need to be good.
- Contracts (for example, between purchasers and providers) are best used to summarise agreement that has already been negotiated elsewhere, not to table points for discussion.
- Implementing evidence may not save money.
- Implementing evidence takes more time than is usually anticipated (Appleby *et al.* 1995 cited by Greenhalgh 1997).

A further project, entitled 'Promoting Action on Clinical Effectiveness' (PACE), has been designed to encourage the implementation of research findings and to promote the development of an evidence-based culture in the National Health Service. Sixteen local 'field sites' in Britain have been established in an attempt to bring clinical practice into line with research evidence (Coulter 1996). The evaluation of this project is also awaited. Finally, many medical schools and continuing medical education programmes now include evidence-based medicine courses and workshops. Incorporating this approach into the application of clinical research within medical education will hopefully lead to a shift in the culture of the practice of health care.

References

Appleby, J., Walsh, K. and Ham, C. (1995) *Acting on the Evidence: A Review of Clinical Effectiveness: Sources of Information, Dissemination and Implementation.* Birmingham: National Association of Health Authorities and Trusts

Ayers, P., Renvoize, T. and Robinson, M. (1995) Clinical guidelines: key decisions for acute service providers. *British Journal of Health Care Management* **1**, 547–51

Cooke, I., Lethaby, A. and Farquhar, C. (1999) 'The effectiveness of antifibrinolytic therapy to reduce heavy menstrual bleeding versus either placebo or any other medication (Cochrane Review)' in: *The Cochrane Library*, Issue 1, 1999. Oxford: Update Software

Coulter, A. (1996) Theory into practice: applying the evidence across the health service. *Baillière's Clin Obstet Gynaecol* **10**, 715–29

Coulter, A., Kelland, J., Peto, V. and Rees, M.C.P. (1995) Treating menorrhagia in primary care. *Int J Technol Assess Health Care* **11**, 454–71

Crowley, P., Chalmers, I. and Keirse, M.J.N.C. (1990) The effects of corticosteroid administration before preterm delivery: an overview of the evidence from controlled trials. *Br J Obstet Gynaecol* **97**, 11–25

Dickersin, K., Scherer, R. and Lefebvre, C. (1995) 'Identifying relevant studies for systematic review' in: I. Chalmers and D.G. Altman (Eds) *Systematic Reviews*. London: BMJ Publishing Group

Dunning, M., McQuary, H. and Milne, R. (1994) Getting a GRiPP. *Health Service Journal* **104**, 18–20

Farquhar, C.M. and Kimble, R. (1996) How do NZ gynaecologists treat menorrhagia? *Aust N Z J Obstet Gynaecol* **36**, 1–4

Field, M.J. and Lohr, I.C.N. (1990) *Clinical Practice Guidelines: Direction of a New Agency*. Washington DC: Institute of Medicine

Greenhalgh, T. (1997) *How to Read a Paper. The Basics of Evidence Based Medicine*. London: BMJ Publishing Group

Grimshaw, J.M. and Russell, I.T. (1993) Effect of clinical guidelines on medical practice. A systematic review of rigorous evaluations. *Lancet* **342**, 1317

James, N.T. (1996) Scientific method and raw data should be considered (letter). *BMJ* **313**, 169–70

Keirse, M.J.N.C. (1984) Obstetrical attitudes to glucocorticoid treatment for lung maturation: time for a change? *Eur J Obstet Gynecol Reprod Biol* **17**, 247–55

Lewis, P.J., de Swiet, M., Boylan, P. and Bulpitt, C.J. (1980) How obstetricians in the UK manage preterm labour. *Br J Obstet Gynaecol* **87**, 574–7

Mann, T. (1996) *Clinical Guidelines: Using Clinical Guidelines to Improve Patient Care Within the NHS*. London: NHS Executive

Oxman, A., Davis, D., Haynes, R.B. *et al.* (1995) No magic bullets: A systematic review of 102 trials of interventions to help health care professionals deliver services more effectively or efficiently. *CMAJ (Ottawa)* **153**, 1423–43

Sackett, D.L. (1996) 'Surveys of self reported reading times of consultants in Oxford, Birmingham, Milton-Keynes, Bristol, Leicester and Glasgow' in: W.M.C. Rosenberg, W.S. Richardson, R.B. Haynes and D.L. Sackett (Eds) *Evidence Based Medicine*. London: Churchill Livingstone

Sackett, D.L. and Haynes, B. (1995) On the need for evidence based medicine. *Evidence-Based Medicine* **1**, 4–5

Sackett, D.L., Haynes, R.B., Guyatt, G.H. and Tugwell, P. (1991) *Clinical Epidemiology: A Basic Science for Clinical Medicine*, 2nd edn. Boston: Little, Brown

Sackett, D.L., Richardson, W.S., Rosenberg, W. and Haynes, R.B. (1996) *Evidence-Based Medicine. How to Practice and Teach EBM*. London: Churchill Livingston

Sacks, H.S., Chalmers, T.C. and Smith, H.J. (1983) Randomisation versus historical assignment in controlled clinical trials. *Am J Med* **309**, 1353–61

9

Audit

Gillian C. Penney

What audit is – and what it is not

The 'official' definition of clinical audit is: 'The systematic and critical analysis of the quality of clinical care, including the procedures used for diagnosis, treatment and care, the associated use of resources and the resulting outcome and quality of life for the patient'.

This definition is taken from *Promoting Clinical Effectiveness* (NHS Executive 1996) and represents a minor modification of the definition first used in the White Paper *Working for Patients* (Department of Health 1989). The definition was originally applied to the term 'medical' audit. During the intervening years between the two NHS publications, it has been applied to the broader term 'clinical' audit. This change reflects an acknowledgement that audit should be a multi-disciplinary activity. The definition conveys that clinical audit involves systematic (structured) and critical (peer review) appraisal of both the process and the outcome of healthcare interventions – with attention to resource use (efficiency).

Confusion over which evaluation exercises constitute 'clinical audit' and which constitute 'clinical research' remains common. Richard Smith, the Editor of the *British Medical Journal*, has succinctly summarised the difference as: 'research is concerned with discovering the right thing to do; audit with ensuring that the thing is done right' (Smith 1992). In other words, the purpose of research is to determine if clinical interventions (whether for diagnosis or treatment) are effective and the purpose of audit is to determine, and to maximise, the extent to which effective interventions are successfully adopted into clinical practice.

Any exercise designed to determine whether a treatment is better than no treatment or whether one treatment is better than another is *not* audit – it is research. Any exercise designed to determine the extent to which a treatment of proven effectiveness is being used in a given clinical setting is audit.

Clinical audit and clinical effectiveness

Clinical effectiveness has been defined as: 'the use of specific clinical interventions which, when deployed in the field for a particular patient or population, do what they are intended to do – i.e. maintain and improve health and secure the greatest possible health gain from the available resources' (NHS Executive 1996).

This definition means that clinical effectiveness involves the use of interventions which combine efficacy (they have been shown to work in the context of research studies), appropriateness (they also work in the real world of patients and populations) and efficiency (or cost effectiveness).

Promoting clinical effectiveness (the use of interventions possessing the attributes outlined above and the rejection of interventions lacking these attributes) is the aim of a major current initiative of the UK NHS Executive. Clinical audit is viewed as a fundamental component of this initiative. The principal role of audit within the clinical effectiveness initiative is to monitor current practice and to verify that change is occurring. However, well-conducted audit has a dual role: not only can it monitor change in practice but the process of audit itself, with feedback of results to participants, can serve as a mechanism to promote change.

Types and styles of clinical audit

Critical incident or adverse event audit

Confidential Enquiries into Maternal Deaths (CEMD) were introduced in the UK in 1952 and typify one style of audit. This approach, known as 'critical incident' or 'adverse event' audit involves the identification of patients where an 'adverse event' (in this case, death) has occurred. The management of the identified cases is then reviewed, perhaps somewhat subjectively, by a panel of experts in order to identify substandard care and to learn lessons for the future. The Department of Health publishes reports on CEMD covering all the UK countries on a three-yearly basis. At the time of writing, the most recent report covered the years 1994–96 (Department of Health 1998).

This adverse event style of audit has subsequently been applied to other subject areas. The National Confidential Enquiry into Peri-operative Deaths (NCEPOD) published its first report in 1989. This enquiry covers the UK (with the exception of Scotland) and aims to include all deaths in hospital within 30 days of a surgical procedure (excluding maternal deaths). The third report of the NCEPOD (published in September 1994) was of particular relevance to gynaecologists as it included an appraisal of deaths following hysterectomy. This report was subsequently summarised for gynaecologists in a review article (Tindall 1994).

The review reflected on the aims of the NCEPOD, which are to examine clinical practice and identify remediable factors and highlighted the incompleteness of the audit, with a rate of return of enquiry forms of 60% by surgeons and 61% by anaesthetists. Despite this incomplete coverage, the NCEPOD review of deaths following hysterectomy identified a number of recurring elements of substandard care. Low use of prophylaxis for deep vein thrombosis, poor attention to postoperative fluid balance and surgeons tackling operations with which they were unfamiliar emerged as particular areas of concern.

A final example of an adverse event audit is the Confidential Enquiry into Stillbirths and Deaths in Infancy (CESDI). At the time of writing, the most recent annual report of CESDI was the fourth, published in 1997 (CESDI 1997). Following the model of the other adverse event audits, CESDI aims to identify cases in which the adverse event of death has occurred. It covers late abortions, stillbirths and deaths in the first year of life. Each year, CESDI selects a subset of these deaths (representing a group where remediable factors seem likely to be found) for detailed confidential enquiry. In the fourth report, this subset comprised 'intrapartum-related deaths among mature, normally formed babies'. Substandard care was identified in relation to 78% of these deaths. Over 70% of the instances of substandard care occurred during labour (with 19% relating to antepartum care and 11% to postpartum care) and over 75% of the instances related to the practice of obstetricians and hospital midwives (the main providers of intrapartum care). The main problem identified was the assessment of fetal condition by heart-rate monitoring and blood sampling.

Topic- or criterion-based audit

An alternative style of audit, described by Charles Shaw (then of the King's Fund) has been termed 'topic-' or 'criterion-based' audit (Shaw 1992). This approach follows the steps of the now classic audit cycle (Figure 9.1).

The fundamental differences between the traditional, adverse event style of audit and this more contemporary approach are as follows:

- In adverse event audit, quality of care is assessed, somewhat subjectively, by expert panels. In contrast, in criterion-based audit, care is assessed more objectively against previously agreed, explicit 'criteria for good quality care'.

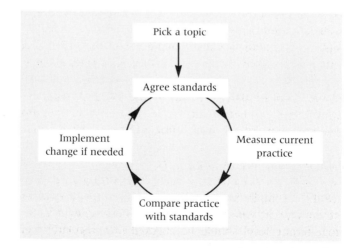

Figure 9.1 The audit cycle

- The reviews of care undertaken in a criterion-based audit are objective and structured, so they can be undertaken by non-expert audit assistants. This means that larger numbers of case records can be reviewed than would be possible within the expert panel approach of an adverse event audit.

Step-by-step guide to criterion-based audit

Criterion-based audit is, in general, the most suitable approach for small audit exercises at the level of the individual hospital or district. The remainder of this chapter is devoted to providing a step-by-step guide to criterion-based audit plus an illustrative example of a completed audit of this type.

Step 1. Pick a topic

As a general rule of thumb, the narrower an audit topic, the greater the likelihood of success. For example, an individual or small group of colleagues would be better conducting an audit of 'confirmation of ovulation among women presenting with infertility' rather than 'the management of infertility' or of 'provision of contraception following induced abortion' rather than 'the management of induced abortion'.

The choice of topic will be largely dictated by the interests of the instigating clinicians, but a number of pointers should be borne in mind:

- The topic should be important in terms of its impact on patient well-being and/or its consumption of health service resources.
- Audit of the topic should be feasible. Feasibility is more likely if:
  - a sufficient research evidence base exists relating to the topic
  - there is a general consensus relating to the topic which is presented in the literature and acceptable to the participants
  - the topic is amenable to the application of objective measurement
  - there is some indication that the topic is amenable to change if deficiencies are identified.
- Sufficient resources are available (largely in terms of staff time and/or information systems) to conduct an audit of the scale and scope planned.

The use of the checklist above will enable the intending auditor to draft a proposal justifying the intended audit topic. A formal, written proposal can then be presented to potential collaborators in order to enlist support.

Step 2. Establish criteria for good quality care

An audit criterion is a succinct statement summarising an element of good quality care. For example, in an audit of 'confirmation of ovulation among women presenting with infertility', an audit criterion might be 'a midluteal plasma progesterone level should be checked in a regularly menstruating female as the basic test of ovulation'.

In an audit of 'provision of contraception following induced abortion', a criterion might be 'if the oral contraceptive pill is chosen as the future method of contraception, pill-taking should begin on the day of induced abortion'.

These examples are of audit criteria relating to the process of care. Criteria may also relate to the outcome of care, for example 'in vitro fertilisation (IVF) should achieve a success rate of 15 live births per 100 cycles commenced' or to the structure of services, for example 'gonadotrophins should only be prescribed in units which have access to ultrasound monitoring and oestradiol assays seven days a week'.

In general, it is most satisfactory to focus on process criteria. Process is usually easier to measure than outcome. If the process criteria used are evidence-based, then good performance in terms of process should be reflected in good outcomes. For example, it is advised that contraceptive pill-taking should commence immediately following abortion on the basis of research showing that a majority of women will resume ovulation within 28 days (Cameron and Baird 1988). Thus, if an abortion service achieves a high proportion of patients beginning the contraceptive pill immediately, this should be reflected in a good outcome in terms of a low proportion of women returning for repeat procedures.

In general, audit criteria should be:
- objective and verifiable, and therefore derived from scientific research (or consensus, if research evidence is lacking)
- capable of being measured
- acceptable to all participating clinicians.

Step 3. Agree on the standards to be met

Having agreed on a set of criteria against which the quality of care will be measured, clinicians may want to agree a related set of 'numerical standards' or 'target percentages' to be met. For example, 'among women who choose the oral contraceptive pill as their method of post-abortion contraception, 100% should begin pill-taking on the day of the procedure'.

This step may be regarded as optional. Clinicians may prefer simply to measure practice in relation to the agreed criterion in a first round of audit and then to regard the performance achieved as the standard to be improved upon in a subsequent round. Thus, if it was found that only 75% of regularly menstruating women referred to a hospital clinic for investigation of infertility had their midluteal progesterone measured prior to referral, it might be agreed to accept 'better than 75%' as the numerical standard or target percentage for a subsequent audit period.

Step 4. Measure current practice

Having established criteria against which practice will be assessed (and, if desired, agreed target percentages to be met), the next step is to observe current practice. It may be possible to assess practice retrospectively using routinely collected information. For example, the Human Fertilisation and

Embryology Authority (HFEA) routinely collects data on all IVF cycles under-taken. An individual clinic could, therefore, draw on this information to audit the outcome of care in its own service. More often, it is necessary to collect data, prospectively or retrospectively, specifically for the audit exercise. This may be done by a variety of means:

- by review of individual patient case records
- by a questionnaire survey of patients
- by a questionnaire survey of clinicians, asking them to describe aspects of their own practice.

For example, an assessment of the proportion of relevant women beginning pill-taking immediately after induced abortion might be made by question-naire survey of the women concerned. Conversely, assessment of the propor-tion of regularly menstruating women who had a midluteal plasma progesterone measured as part of the initial investigation of infertility might best be achieved by review of the patients' records.

If a questionnaire approach is chosen, the auditor must be aware of the potentially serious bias which may be introduced should the response rate be poor.

Step 5. Compare practice with the agreed criteria

Following measurement of current practice by the chosen means, the findings must be summarised so as to identify aspects of care which are satisfactory (by measuring up well to the agreed criteria) and for which changes are required. For example, if all women who chose the contraceptive pill following abor-tion were surveyed and all said that they had been provided with a supply of pills while in hospital and had taken their first pill prior to discharge, then it would be agreed that this aspect of care was satisfactory and no change was required. Conversely, if a review of the case records of women referred by their GPs for hospital investigation of infertility revealed that only 40% of those with regular menstrual cycles had had a midluteal progesterone checked prior to referral – it would probably be agreed that change was required.

Step 6. Implement change where indicated

Assuming that the audit reveals some aspects of care which measure up poorly against the agreed criteria, the next step is to promote appropriate change in practice. In choosing approaches which might persuade colleagues to change, it is important first to attempt to determine, for each deficient aspect of practice, the reason for the deficiency. There are five principal expla-nations for care falling short of agreed standards:

- the agreed criterion is invalid or the standard set is unrealistic
- the organisation of care is deficient
- knowledge is inadequate

- skills are inadequate
- attitudes are inappropriate.

Sometimes the explanation for deficiencies may be glaringly obvious but, more often, teasing out the contribution of various causes may be difficult. However, since the purpose of audit is to bring about improvements, this step must be tackled if the exercise is not to have been merely a waste of resources.

This analysis of the reasons for deficiencies in care and of the barriers to change leads to the design of interventions to promote change. Such measures might include:

- checklists (patient-specific reminders) to be completed by the clinician during, or shortly after, a clinical consultation
- the use of clinical guidelines, diagnostic algorithms, treatment protocols, and so on
- feedback to clinicians of audit results, indicating the extent to which current practice departs from the standards set.

Step 7. Repeat measurement of practice to confirm beneficial change

Audit should not be merely a one-off observation of practice, but should include repeat measurement after an appropriate time interval, in order to monitor the extent of change. Knowledge of impending re-audit can, in itself, act as a stimulus to clinicians to introduce changes.

Ideally, an audit exercise should not comprise just the completion of an audit cycle as described above, but should constitute what has been termed an 'audit spiral'. Measurement of practice is repeated on a number of occasions, with revision of criteria and standards if required due to the availability of new evidence. It is to be hoped that such an audit spiral will demonstrate constantly improving standards of care.

Illustrative example of a criterion-based audit: three rounds of audit of the management of induced abortion

An audit of the management of induced abortion was undertaken in Scotland during 1992 and 1993. This formed part of the Gynaecology Audit Project in Scotland (GAPS). Two rounds of prospective, criterion based, case-note review audit were undertaken in ten representative hospitals (Penney *et al.* 1994a). In addition, the outcome of care, from the patients' viewpoint, was assessed by questionnaire survey of women identified through the case-note review exercises (Penney *et al.* 1994b).

Following this national audit, one of the participating hospitals acknowledged that further improvements in abortion care were required. After organisational changes within the gynaecology department, a third round of case-note review and a further questionnaire survey of patients was undertaken within this single hospital. The data collection methods and documentation were identical to those used in the national audit. The results in this one hospital of the successive rounds of this audit are presented here as an illustrative example of an exercise which progressed some way along the audit spiral.

Establishing criteria for good quality care

For the national project, a list of criteria for good quality care relating to induced abortion was agreed by a combination of objective review of contemporary medical literature, panel discussions and a postal survey of all consultant gynaecologists in Scotland (Penney *et al.* 1993). The 13 criteria which were addressed in all three successive rounds of audit in the one study hospital are listed in Table 9.1.

Eleven of the criteria relate to the processes of care provided to individual

---

Table 9.1 Criteria for good quality care agreed among consultant gynaecologists in Scotland and addressed in case-note review audit

Organisation of the service
1 All women requesting abortion should be offered an appointment with a gynaecologist within five days of referral.
2 Induced abortion should be undertaken within seven days of the appointment with the gynaecologist.
3 In the absence of specific medical or social contraindications, women undergoing abortion should be managed as day cases.

Pre-abortion investigations
4 The woman's Rh status should be ascertained and Rh prophylaxis given following abortion, if indicated.
5 Women undergoing abortion should be screened for genital tract infection and treated if indicated.

Methods of abortion
6 Women presenting early in pregnancy (less than nine weeks' gestation) should have the option of surgical or medical abortion.
7 In selecting women undergoing surgical abortion, technique for cervical predilation should be used.
8 All surgical abortions at gestations over ten weeks should be carried out by an experienced gynaecologist (post MRCOG or equivalent).
9 For second-trimester medical abortions, pretreatment with mifepristone reduces the induction-abortion interval.

Post-abortion care
10 Before being discharged, each patient should have agreed a contraceptive plan.
11 Before being discharged, each patient should be offered contraceptive supplies.
12 A follow-up appointment, either at hospital or with the referring doctor, should be given to every patient.
13 The follow-up appointment should be within two weeks of abortion procedure.

---

patients. Two (numbers six and nine) relate to what might be termed the structure of care and to whether or not specific elements of service are available. Results relating to the 11 'process' criteria are expressed in terms of the percentage of patients in whom the criterion was met, whereas results relating to the two 'structure' criteria are expressed simply in terms of whether or not that service was available.

Measuring current practice

During each of the two national audit periods and a three-month local audit period, all women undergoing induced abortion in one gynaecology unit were identified and data relating to the agreed criteria were collected by secretarial audit assistants by transfer of information from case-notes to a review document (Penney *et al.* 1994a).

Each patient was asked by ward staff if she would be willing to participate in a survey about her care. A questionnaire (Penney *et al.* 1994b) was sent to the home address of each consenting woman four weeks post-abortion. It addressed the following topics:

- general satisfaction with care
- provision of emotional support
- provision of contraceptive advice and supplies
- views on the availability of a choice of abortion methods
- follow-up arrangements
- health problems following abortion.

Completed questionnaires were returned to the audit office using a stamped addressed envelope.

Data from the case-note reviews and from the patient questionnaires were entered into a database using Paradox® (Borland) software. Data from the successive rounds of audit were compared and statistical significance tested by chi-squared analysis.

Comparing practice with the agreed criteria (and with practice during the previous audit periods)

During the three-month local audit period, 389 consecutive patients were identified. Of these, 114 (29%) completed the patient questionnaire. Table 9.2 summarises the results of the case-note review relating to the 13 criteria. Results relating to this series of 389 patients can be compared with those relating to the 100 and 209 patients studied in the same hospital during the two national audit periods.

Significant improvements (at the $P < 0.05$ level) had occurred since the second national audit period in relation to six of the 13 criteria:

- Patients seen within five days of referral rose from 26% to 38%.
- Cases having genital tract bacteriology swabs taken prior to abortion rose from 6% to 63%.

Table 9.2   Results in relation to 13 agreed audit criteria in three successive rounds of case-note review audit

Criterion	Element of care	National audit year 1 (n = 100)[a]	National audit year 2 (n = 209)[a]	Local audit (n = 389)[a]
1	Percentage of cases seen within five days of referral	29	26	38
2	Percentage of procedures undertaken within seven days of clinic attendance	89	86	90
3	Percentage of patients managed as day cases	63	82[b]	82
4	Percentage of cases where rhesus status recorded	99	95	100
5	Percentage of cases where genital tract bacteriology swabs taken	14	6	63[b]
6	Early medical abortion service available	Yes	Yes	Yes
7	Percentage of high risk abortions (>10 weeks surgical gestation and/ or age <17 years) having cervical priming	69 (18/26)	86 (30/35)	94 (24/26)
8	Percentage of surgical abortions at >10 weeks performed by senior registrar or above	54 (12/22)	75 (21/28)	92 (24/26)
9	Mifepristone priming in use prior to midtrimester medical abortion	Yes	Yes	Yes
10	Percentage of cases where contraceptive plan recorded	57	46	95[b]
11	Percentage of cases provided with contraceptive method by hospital staff	16	6	45[b]
12	Percentage of cases where follow-up plan recorded	25	52b	76[b]
13	Percentage of cases where follow-up within two week advised	4	35b	44[b]

[a] These figures represent the performance of a single hospital in each audit period – the local figures from a national audit in years 1 and 2); [b] Significant improvement at $P < 0.05$ (χ^2 test)

- Patients for whom a future contraceptive plan was recorded rose from 46% to 95%.
- Patients provided with contraceptive supplies by hospital staff rose from 6% to 45%.
- Patients for whom a follow-up plan was recorded rose from 52% to 76%.
- Patients being offered follow-up within the recommended interval of two weeks rose from 35% to 44%.

Table 9.3 summarises the responses of the 114 women who returned outcome questionnaires for comparison with those of the 61 women from this hospital (20% of those eligible) who responded during the national audit. Significant changes (at the $P < 0.05$ level) had occurred in relation to seven of 12 elements of care addressed:

- Patients indicating that they felt their decision had been right for them rose from 78% to 94%.
- Those reporting that they received enough emotional support from hospital staff rose from 65% to 86%.
- Those indicating that contraception had been discussed with them by hospital staff rose from 78% to 96%.
- Those indicating that contraceptive supplies were offered to them prior to discharge rose from 30% to 77%.
- Those who were aware of emergency contraception rose from 66% to 88%.
- Those reporting that a follow-up appointment had been arranged for them rose from 46% to 84%.
- Those indicating that they felt the follow-up appointment was worthwhile rose from 78% to 93%.

The low response rates obtained in the patient survey element of this audit highlight the problem of such an approach. Nevertheless, there is still some validity in examining change over time using such an approach, as it is likely that women sharing similar characteristics would have responded in each time period.

The Gynaecology Audit Project in Scotland prompted open and objective discussions among clinicians about abortion care in Scottish hospitals and a majority of gynaecologists reported that they had changed or reconsidered aspects of their practice in response to this audit exercise (Penney and Templeton 1995). In the hospital described here, local results within the multi-centre audit enabled clinicians to acknowledge deficiencies in their local service. In response to the audit findings, reorganisation within the gynaecology department resulted in the formation of dedicated pregnancy counselling clinics and in the appointment of two nurses with responsibility for ensuring the smooth running of the abortion service and for the provision of contraceptive advice and supplies.

Table 9.3 Results in relation to patients' perceptions of care in two audit periods

Criterion	Element of care	National audit (n = 61)[a]	Local audit (n = 114)[a]
1	Percentage satisfied or very satisfied with care provided by doctors	88	84
2	Percentage satisfied or very satisfied with care provided by nursing and ancillary staff	92	93
3	Percentage indicating they had enough time and help in reaching their decision	78	90
4	Percentage indicating that (at four weeks post-abortion) they felt their decision was right	78	94[b]
5	Percentage indicating that overall they received enough emotional support from hospital staff	65	86[b]
6	Percentage indicating that contraception was discussed with them by hospital staff	78	96[b]
7	Percentage indicating that contraceptive supplies had been offered to them by hospital staff	30	77[b]
8	Percentage who had adopted a contraceptive method at four weeks post-abortion	88	88
9	Percentage indicating awareness of emergency contraception	66	88[b]
10	Percentage reporting that a follow-up appointment had been arranged	46	84[b]
11	Percentage indicating that they felt follow-up was worthwhile	78	93[b]
12	Percentage reporting post-abortion health problems	27	20

[a] These figures represent the performance of a single hospital in each audit period – the local figures from a national audit during period one; [b] Significant improvement at $P < 0.05$ (χ^2 test)

Local staff undertook to monitor the effects of these organisational changes by means of a repeat audit resourced using local audit funds. It is encouraging that measurable changes in the quality of care, as assessed by both case-note review and patient survey, were demonstrable. Although response rates to the patient survey were, understandably, low on both occasions, it was felt that comparisons between the two time periods were valid.

This audit exercise, undertaken within a single hospital and using local resources, demonstrates the usefulness of clinical audit both in prompting changes in practice and in monitoring the impact of such changes. It is encouraging that a programme of audit initiated as part of a national exercise was continued at the local level – thus allowing progression along the audit spiral.

References

Cameron, I.T. and Baird, D.T. (1988) The return to ovulation following early abortion: a comparison between vacuum aspiration and prostaglandin. *Acta Endocrinologica (Copenhagen)* **118**, 161–7

CESDI (1997) *4th Annual Report*. London: Maternal and Child Health Research Consortium

Department of Health (1998) *Why Mothers die. Report on Confidential Enquiries into Maternal Deaths in the United Kingdom 1994–1996*. London: TSO

Department of Health (1989) *Working for Patients. Medical Audit*. London: HMSO

NHS Executive (1996) *Promoting Clinical Effectiveness: A Framework for Action in and Through the NHS*. London: NHS Executive

Penney, G.C. and Templeton, A. (1995) Impact of a national audit project on gynaecologists in Scotland. *Quality in Health Care* **4**, 37–9

Penney, G.C., Glasier, A. and Templeton, A. (1993) Agreeing criteria for audit of the management of induced abortion: an approach by national consensus survey. *Quality in Health Care* **2**, 167–9

Penney, G.C., Glasier, A. and Templeton, A. (1994a) A multi-centre, criterion-based audit of the management of induced abortion in Scotland. *BMJ* **309**, 15–8

Penney, G.C., Glasier, A. and Templeton, A. (1994b) Patients' views on abortion care in Scottish hospitals. *Health Bull* **52**, 431–8

Shaw, C.D. (1992) 'Criterion based audit' in R. Smith (Ed.) *Audit in Action*, pp. 122–8. London: BMJ Publishing Group

Smith, R. (1992) Audit and research. *BMJ* **305**, 905–6

Tindall, V.R. (1994) The national confidential enquiry into perioperative deaths. *Br J Obstet Gynaecol* **101**, 468–70

## 10

Clinical trials

Richard B. Johanson

Archie Cochrane suggested that we should aim to implement those forms of care which have been shown in properly designed evaluations to be effective (Cochrane 1972). A number of considerations need to be addressed if an evaluation is going to be deemed *properly designed*.

- It is essential that properly designed evaluations consider all important outcomes. For example, biochemical outcomes are not usually considered as important to patients as clinical, psychological and psychosocial outcomes. The size of the study (n) will depend on the primary or principle outcome chosen.
- Not only is it important to know the expected benefits and potential harms of an intervention, but cost-effectiveness information will also need to be obtained. In his examination of the debate surrounding the benefits and harms of prostatectomy for benign prostatic hyperplasia, Wennberg points out the 'scandalous' fact that, while over 350 000 prostatectomies were performed annually in the USA, by 1989 fewer than 400 patients had been followed systematically to study the 'main effect' outcome: the effect of the operation on symptom status (Wennberg 1990). This example illustrates the real economic costs of a surgical intervention which, at that time, had been subjected to very little properly designed evaluation (and which might even cause more harm than good).
- The results of the evaluation should show how large and how precise was the treatment effect (Guyatt *et al.* 1993).

Presenting data in this way will facilitate decision analysis (Hirsh *et al.* 1970): the process of joint planning of care which has become a fundamental aspect of current clinical effectiveness programmes.

The evolution of clinical trials

The accepted current 'gold standard' in terms of properly designed evaluations is the randomised controlled trial (RCT). This design, if properly undertaken, minimises bias and allows small, but clinically significant, differences in benefit and harm to be detected (provided n is large enough). It may also allow valid inferences about 'cause and effect', depending on a number of factors (Campbell and Machin 1993). There have been and still are numerous examples in the literature of problems associated with other clinical trial designs.

'Uncontrolled' trials

When innovations in medicine occur, they are often enthusiastically adopted by avant-garde clinicians and tried out on a few patients in an uncontrolled trial. To give the innovative treatment a reasonable chance of success, one might subconsciously select less seriously ill patients. Consequently, regardless of the treatment's real value, it is likely that such a selected group of patients will do well, compared with the generally accepted management. A good example of the mistakes that occur with intuitive research was the widespread adoption, on the basis of physiological and pharmacological observations, of a specific antidysrhythmic drug for use after myocardial infarction (Morganroth *et al.* 1990). Subsequent RCTs found that these drugs increase, rather than decrease, the risk of death in such patients (Echt *et al.* 1991).

To avoid this distorted view of therapy, most researchers recognised the need for a 'control' group. However, because many clinicians assume that the new treatment will invariably be better, there has been a reluctance to assign patients randomly. Instead, it was preferred to assign 'historical' or 'concurrent' controls (patients with the same condition, matched as far as possible for major prognostic indicators).

'Historical' controls

The most common way of obtaining a control group that seemed acceptable was to compare retrospectively one's current patients on the new treatment with previous patients who had received standard treatment (historical controls). There are two major sources of bias using this approach: 'patient selection' and 'the experimental environment' (Pocock 1984). The 'historical' group may not have the same narrow inclusion criteria and may be from a different source/environment. In addition, it is likely that the quality of recorded data for the historical group will be poorer and it is possible that other aspects of ancillary patient care may have improved. There may also be a tendency to exclude from the analysis more patients on the 'new' treatment than in the 'historical' control group on the basis that the treatment received was not protocol based (and therefore 'invalid'). The net effect is a bias, most frequently in favour of the new treatment.

Grage and Zelen showed how several studies with historical controls (involving over 1000 patients) extolled the value of an invasive new treatment of liver metastases, while the only RCT showed no advantage (Grage and Zelen 1982). Similarly, based on 'historical' data, high concentration oxygen therapy was used for preterm babies, but only after pioneering RCT work did it become clear that this was the cause of infants' blindness due to retrolental fibroplasia (Lanman *et al.* 1954).

'Concurrent' controls

Various methods of obtaining a concurrent control group have been tried. Smithells *et al.*, believing that randomisation was unethical in a high-risk group of women who had experienced a previous neural tube defect, allowed women who did not want to take supplements (and also some women who were already pregnant) to be part of their untreated control group (Smithells *et al.* 1980). They found that multi-vitamin preparations were potentially 'useful' in preventing neural tube defects. The study was seriously flawed (women who chose to take vitamins probably represented a selected group, perhaps with a more affluent or health-conscious diet, who were therefore at low risk of having a further abnormal pregnancy), with resulting poor information for patients and a significant delay in carrying out the definitive study. Indeed, ethics committees were unwilling to deprive patients of this potentially 'useful' treatment, making it difficult to carry out the trial which later showed that folic acid was the effective part of the multi-vitamin cocktail (MRC Vitamin Study Research Group 1991).

RCTs

Ethics of randomisation

Chalmers argued that 'the only way to avoid the distorting influences of uncontrolled trials is to begin randomisation with the first patient' (Chalmers 1972). Randomisation avoids the problems of bias and over-optimistic expectations of new therapy. It also gives patients a 50% chance of receiving the more effective treatment, whichever one that is. It is particularly valuable when a new therapy is expensive (when it is also the 'fairest' way of giving each patient an equal chance of receiving the expensive treatment). It remains ethical even when the new treatment is cheap, as experience has shown that many new treatments are not better (Gilbert *et al.* 1977) and that a significant proportion will cause harm (Chalmers *et al.* 1989). 'Uncertainty' about the benefits of a new treatment is a generally accepted starting point for an RCT. It has been well argued that 'equipoise' has a more precise meaning and reflects the fact that knowledge comes in degrees and that 'value' should also be entered into the equation (particularly when judging the trade-off of benefits and side effects) (Edwards *et al.* 1998).

Random allocation and 'blinding'

In the simplest design, patients are randomly allocated to one of two groups (conventionally known as 'treatment' and 'control'). This ensures that there will be no systematic difference between intervention groups in factors, known and unknown, that may affect outcome (Sibbald and Roland 1998). A range of other random allocation designs are possible, including 'cross-over' and designs where the randomisation is not necessarily 1:1 (Pocock 1984).

If the groups are large enough, the 'treatment' and 'control' should be similar in all respects at the start of the trial. This will include a balance of those variables considered to be prognostic. In smaller trials, it may be necessary to stratify according to several characteristics or the minimisation method (Pocock 1984). It is essential that the investigator should not know what the allocation will be. Allocation assigned on the basis of 'date of birth' or 'date of presentation' is likely to result in unbalanced selective recruitment. Even allocation using 'sealed opaque envelopes' has a potential for bias if envelopes are opened and not used or become 'lost'. Randomisation should ideally be by computer allocation, or via a central telephone link.

Wherever possible, both patients and triallists should remain unaware of which treatment is given until the study is completed (a 'double-blind' study). While feasible for drug trials, this design clearly would be impossible for surgical studies. Indeed, evaluation of therapy in normal clinical practice, where both the patient and the investigator know the actual treatment, has been termed 'pragmatic' (Russell 1995). The alternative research scenario, where only 'ideal' patients are included and operated on in 'ideal' circumstances, has been described as 'fastidious'. 'Pragmatic' trials have the advantage of having more potential for generalisation than 'fastidious' trials (Russell 1995). Wherever possible, the outcome assessment should be undertaken by an observer 'blind' to the original treatment allocation.

Meta-analysis of controlled trials shows that failure to conceal random allocation and the absence of blinded assessment yield exaggerated estimates of treatment effects (Schulz *et al.* 1995).

Description of eligible and included patients
Information on the number and characteristics of eligible patients who do not wish to enter an RCT should be collected, as this may be important in the assessment of the potential for generalisation (Charlson and Horwitz 1984).

All patients entered into a study should be accounted for in the report (including 'drop-outs'). Follow-up should be complete.

Treatment and analysis of the two groups
Patients in both sides of the study should be managed identically in all respects excepting the experimental treatment.

Patients should be analysed within the group to which they were allocated, irrespective of whether they experienced the intended intervention (intention-to-treat analysis). Although some find this concept intuitively difficult to accept, this is fundamentally important. The alternative would be to analyse on the basis of treatment received. This can be explained with an example from clinical research in obstetrics. Assisted vaginal delivery can be carried out either with a vacuum extractor or with forceps. It is well known that failure with the vacuum extractor is more likely than with forceps. Some of the women in this group will have their delivery completed by forceps, others will have a caesarean section. Morbidity is greatest after instrumental delivery where multiple attempts at delivery were made. If, therefore, we included the women who had a failed vacuum delivery completed by forceps in the forceps group, we will be biasing the study against forceps. They are, therefore, kept in the group into which they were originally allocated for the purpose of the primary analysis.

Designing a new trial:
a worked example of an obstetric RCT

Developing the question

Variations in surgical practice are common. One obstetric example currently receiving prominence is the best management of anal injury resulting from a vaginal birth (third degree tear). Two different methods for repair exist and each has its proponents. Traditionally, the sphincter muscle has been repaired with an 'end-to-end' juxtaposition and anastomosis of the torn anal sphincter muscle. The new method of repair (or 'intervention') involves an overlapping technique. This is particularly important because of the possibility of an adverse long-term 'outcome that matters' (faecal incontinence at three months). This question encompasses the 'principle objective' or 'hypothesis' in terms of three aspects:

- participants
- intervention and control care
- outcome measures.

Systematic review, professional survey and consumer involvement
Systematic review

It is vitally important at this stage to search for a systematic review of the literature to ensure that no-one else has looked at this question. The first place to start would be *The Cochrane Library* with its database of systematic reviews (see Chapter 6). If a systematic review has not yet been undertaken, this will need to be done.

Professional survey

It would also be valuable to obtain a picture of current obstetric practice and of interest in participation in a multi-centre study. This information should be sought in a professional survey.

Consumer involvement

Consumer input at this stage is essential, not only in designing the study, but also in encouraging women to participate. The manner in which consumers are involved will vary, from 'consultation' through to 'joint lead-investigator'. Input should be sought on all aspects of the study and, specifically, in terms of determining the principle end-point and other outcome measures (and the timing of the assessment of outcome/s) and in developing questionnaires.

Focus group and in-depth interview techniques are valuable. It is surprising how few studies have involved long-term follow-up to include 'outcomes that matter to the participant'.

Sample size and statistics

From the literature review (or pilot studies), it should be possible to estimate the potential difference one might expect to see between treatments (in terms of the principle end-point). In the study on third degree tears being discussed, a difference of even 5% in terms of incontinence might be deemed both clinically and statistically significant. If one knows the baseline figures for standard treatment (e.g. 20%) and if one is hoping to undertake a study sufficiently large to detect a modest improvement (e.g. to 15%), then the sample size can be calculated. Any trial should be sufficiently large to detect the size of difference which would influence clinical practice. At the very least, it should be sufficiently powerful in combination (by meta-analysis) with other trials that are under way (Lilford and Thornton 1992).

Conventionally, the power is set at 80% (which means that there is a 20% chance of missing a difference that is actually there ('type II error' or $\beta = 0.20$). Additionally, the conventional statistical significance level chosen is 5%, which means that there is a 5% chance of finding a difference (simply by chance) that does not exist in reality (probability of 'type I error' or $\alpha = 0.05$). Given these parameters, the sample size in our example can be calculated (using commercially available software) to be 900 in each group. Clearly, if one wished to detect a smaller difference, or if one wanted a larger power or higher level of significance, the study would need to be larger. This method of calculating power is based on the standard view that a false positive result (type I error) is more serious than a false negative result (type II error). This approach is challenged by those who promote the use of decision theory, where the size of a study will be related directly to the size of difference regarded as important (Lilford and Thornton 1992).

Power calculations can also be based on continuous data. If the principle end-point is measured on a continuous scale of severity, baseline mean and standard deviation values for the population should be established. The sample size is calculated from the differences of effect size, that is the expected difference between the two means ('control' and 'treatment', divided by the – assumed – common standard deviation). This means that, for a given sample size, the smaller the standard deviation, the smaller the difference between the means that can be detected.

It is also possible to estimate sample size simply on the basis of likely size of effect (Cohen 1988). This is valuable when the investigator does not have data on baseline values of mean and standard deviation. Cohen (1988) defines a small effect size to be 0.2, a medium effect size to be 0.5 and a large effect size to be 0.8. With 50 participants in each half of a trial, the power to detect these effects would be 17%, 71% and 98%, respectively.

In summary, the overall message about sample size is 'the smaller the difference you wish to detect, the larger the study needs to be'.

Ethics committee approval and the data monitoring committee

Ethics committees will follow BMA guidelines, among others. When evaluating an RCT protocol for obstetric care they will also want to see that the recommendations agreed by the National Childbirth Trust (NCT) and the Association for Improvements in the Maternity Services (AIMS) are being followed (NCT/AIMS 1997). A trial becomes ethical when both the clinician and the participant are in equipoise; that is, they expect the utility to be the same with both treatments (Lilford and Thornton 1992; see Chapter 17). The protocol, questionnaires and information sheets will need to be prepared prior to obtaining ethics committee approval.

Ethics committees will, in some studies, expect to see in place a 'data monitoring committee'. This committee may be required to carry out one or more interim analyses. Where the new treatment is worse (for example, due to side effects) or dramatically better, then the committee will recommend termination of the study, so as not to further disadvantage participants receiving the less beneficial treatment (UK Collaborative ECMO Trial Group 1996). Fayers *et al.* (1997) recommend using a Bayesian approach (see below) to monitoring RCTs. They suggest that this will help to ensure that studies should only stop early when the results are sufficiently conclusive (i.e. that sufficient data have been collected to convince even 'sceptical' clinicians). See Chapter 17 for more detailed discussions of ethics and ethics committees.

Design into reality

Having developed the question, undertaken the relevant background work, obtained statistical advice and ethical committee approval, it should now be possible to obtain interest from other possible collaborators. At this point, the protocol should have reached a suitable stage of development to be submitted as a grant proposal.

Alternative RCT designs

Patient preference trials

Some patients who agree to participate in an RCT do so in an effort to receive the new treatment. Llewellyn-Thomas *et al.* showed that over 90% of patients who agreed to participate in a clinical trial had a preference for the new treatment, compared to 62% of the whole study sample (Llewellyn-Thomas *et al.* 1991). The allocation of a patient to the old treatment may reduce their motivation for compliance or continued participation. Strong patient preferences for 'keyhole' gall bladder surgery meant that only 8.6% of eligible patients (those in 'equipoise') were recruited to a trial comparing this 'new' treatment to standard open cholecystectomy (Plaisier *et al.* 1994). Brewin and Bradley suggested a design to increase patient recruitment to clinical trials, called the partially randomised patient preference trial (Bradley 1988). This design allows patients with a strong preference to receive their chosen treatment while the remainder are randomised. Although the data generated by the preference groups will inherently reflect selection bias, they will, by comparison with the data obtained from the randomised cohort, enable an estimate of the size of motivational effect to be calculated. Henshaw *et al.* (1993) carried out a patient preference partially randomised comparison of medical and surgical termination of pregnancy. The randomised cohort evaluation demonstrated that both treatments were equally effective; however, acceptability was higher in the preference groups. These become important issues when making decisions with patients in clinical practice.

McPherson *et al.* (1997) have acknowledged the importance of estimating the size of preference effects. The challenge is to then disentangle the main physical effect of treatment.

Zelen randomisation method

Zelen (1979) suggested that one of the principal reasons why clinical investigators decline to participate in randomised studies is that they believe that the 'patient–physician relation' is compromised. He observed that physicians may find it difficult to tell patients that they do not know which treatment is best. He proposed a system whereby half the patients are randomised to the current standard 'best' therapy. They do not have to give consent. The other half are randomised to the 'new' treatment. After assignation, the patient gives consent. If he/she declines to participate, then they simply go back to receiving the current standard 'best' therapy. This method has been used in obstetric research, for example, the Gardosi birth-cushion trial (Gardosi *et al.* 1989).

Cluster randomised trials

Trials which randomise intact social groups, or clusters, to different interventions are becoming increasingly common (Donner 1998). They have become widely used in the past two decades for the evaluation of health care and educational strategies, where medical practices, schools or even entire communities are often selected as the unit of randomisation. The members of the units cannot be regarded as statistically independent, so these designs tend to be less efficient than designs which randomise individuals. As such, the justification for choosing this method must always be explicit. The situations where this method would be appropriate can be divided into those where it is not possible to separate the intervention from the individual (e.g. an advertising campaign to stop smoking) or where individual randomisation would be scientifically inappropriate (e.g. because of 'contamination' between individuals in the study). The World Health Organization antenatal care trial, currently under way, is an example of such a design. It aims to compare traditional antenatal care with a more limited 'evidence-based' antenatal care package. Clearly, it would be impossible to run both forms of care in the same clinics. The cluster randomisation design is essential for logistic and administrative convenience. It also reduces the 'treatment contamination' that is likely to occur under individual randomisation. Although the end-points are measured in individual outcomes, power calculations have to be undertaken on the basis of the number of clusters in the study. Various statistical models are being developed for analysis of outcome data from cluster randomisation trials and informed advice should be sought.

Bayesian trials

Bayesian methods have been proposed as a way to provide useful information in situations where diseases are rare and benefits modest and where currently conceived clinical trials will have little to contribute (because the sample size will never be achievable). Using the Bayesian approach, all available data are used to calculate probabilities. These can then be used in decision analyses in clinical practice (Lilford et al. 1995). Clinicians 'prior' beliefs or expectations are obtained. The quality of available evidence will affect the 'objectivity' of the 'priors'. Priors based on trial data will be less subjective than those based simply on the opinions of experts. The purpose of the trial is to alter that belief according to the strength of the evidence. Trial data can be analysed as they become available, a so-called 'open' trial. It is possible to measure the amended clinical prior belief ('posterior distribution') and then combine these with the randomised results to calculate the probabilities of different sizes of treatment effect. Although incorrect results can be produced, Lilford et al. (1995) believe strongly that 'a decision taken on the basis of a posterior belief that includes evidence from an RCT however small, is more likely to be correct than a decision based simply on a prior belief with no evidence from such a trial. Any randomised evidence is better than none'.

Conclusions

We should aim for our research to be properly designed. There should be a focus on consumer outcomes, with results showing treatment effect size and precision. In order to feed into health policy equations and decision analysis, cost-effectiveness should also be measured. A wide variety of RCT designs has been developed. The randomised controlled trial should be considered as the 'gold standard' for evaluating both established and new interventions.

Acknowledgements
Peter Jones (Professor of Statistics, Keele University), Chris Kettle (Research Midwife 'MOMS' trial), Gill Gyte (Cochrane Consumer Network) and Richard Lilford (Director, West Midlands Research and Development) for their helpful comments and Nicola Leighton (Research Assistant) for preparing the manuscript. Richard Johanson's Clinical Trials work is supported by a five-year West Midlands Research and Development grant.

References

Bradley, C. (1988) Clinical trials – time for a paradigm shift? *Diabet Med* **5**, 107–9

Campbell, M.J. and Machin, D. (1993) *Medical Statistics; A Common Sense Approach*, 2nd edn. Chichester: John Wiley & Sons

Chalmers, I., Enkin, M. and Keirse, M.J.N.C. (1989) 'Forms of care that reduced negative outcomes of pregnancy and childbirth' in: I. Chalmers, M. Enkin and M.J.N.C. Keirse (Eds) *Effective Care in Pregnancy and Childbirth*, pp. 1471–6. Oxford: Oxford University Press

Chalmers, T.C. (1972) Randomization and coronary artery surgery. *Ann Thorac Surg* **14**, 323–7

Charlson, M.E. and Horwitz, R.I. (1984) Applying results of randomised trials to clinical practice: impact of losses before randomisation. *BMJ* **289**, 1281–4

Cochrane, A.L. (1972) *Effectiveness and Efficiency: Random Reflections on Health Services*. London: Nuffield Provincial Hospitals Trust

Cohen, J. (1988) *Statistical Power Analysis for the Behavioural Sciences*. New Jersey: Lawrence Erlbaum Associates

Donner, A. (1998) Some aspects of the design and analysis of cluster randomization trials. *Applied Statistics* **47**, 95–113

Echt, D.S., Liebson, P.R., Mitchell, B. *et al.* (1991) Mortality and morbidity in patients receiving encainide, flecainide, or placebo: the Cardiac Arrhythmia Suppression Trial. *New Engl J Med* **324**, 781–8

Edwards, S.J.C., Lilford, R.J., Braunholtz, D.A., Jackson, J.C., Hewison, J. and Thornton, J. (1998) 'Ethics of randomised controlled trials' in: N. Black, J. Brazier, J. Fitzpatrick and B. Reeves (Eds) *Health Service Research Methods*, pp. 98–107. London: BMJ Publishing Group

Fayers, P.M., Ashby, D. and Parmar, M.K.B. (1997) Tutorial in Biostatistics: Bayesian data monitoring in clinical trials. *Stat Med* **16**, 1413–30

Gardosi, J., Hutson, N. and B-Lynch, C. (1989) Randomised, controlled trial of squatting in the second stage of labour. *Lancet* **ii**, 74–7

Gilbert, J.P., McPeek, B. and Mosteller, F. (1977) Statistics and ethics in surgery and anaesthesia. *Science* **198**, 689

Grage, T.B. and Zelen, M. (1982) The controlled randomized trial in the evaluation of cancer treatment – the dilemma and alternative designs. *UICC Technical Report Series* **70**, 23–47

Guyatt, G.H., Sackett, D.L. and Cook, D.J. (1993) Users' Guides to the Medical Literature; how to use an article about therapy or prevention; are the results of the study valid? *JAMA* **270**, 2598–601

Henshaw, R.C., Naji, S.A., Russell, I.T. and Templeton, A.A. (1993) Comparison of medical abortion with surgical vacuum aspiration: women's preferences and acceptability of treatment. *BMJ* **307**, 714–17

Hirsh, J., Cade, J.F. and O'Sullivan, E.F. (1970) Clinical experience with anticoagulant therapy during pregnancy. *BMJ* **1**, 270–3

Lanman, J.T., Guy, L.P. and Dancis, J. (1954) Retrolental fibroplasia and oxygen therapy. *JAMA* **155**, 223–5

Lilford, R.J., Thornton, J.G. and Braunholtz, D. (1995) Clinical trials and rare diseases: a way out of a conundrum. *BMJ* **311**, 1621–5

Lilford, R.J. and Thornton, J.D. (1992) Decision logic in medical practice. *J R Coll Physicians Lond* **26**, 400–12

Llewellyn-Thomas, H.A., McGreal, M.J., Thiel, E.C., Fine, S. and Erlichman, C. (1991) Patients' willingness to enter clinical trials: measuring the association with perceived benefit and preference for decision participation. *Soc Sci Med* **32**, 35–42

McPherson, K., Britton, A., R. and Wennberg, J.E. (1997) Are randomized controlled trials controlled? Patient preferences and unblind trials. *J Roy Soc Med* **90**, 652–6

Morganroth, J., Bigger, J.T.J. and Anderson, J.L. (1990) Treatment of ventricular arrhythmia by United States cardiologists: a survey before the Cardiac Arrhythmia Suppression Trial results were available. *Am J Cardiol* **65**, 40–8

MRC Vitamin Study Research Group (1991) Prevention of neural tube defects. Results of the MRC vitamin study. *Lancet* **338**, 131–7

NCT/AIMS (National Childbirth Trust and Association for Improvements in the Maternity Services), (1997) *A Charter for Ethical Research in Maternity Care.* London: NCT and AIMS.

Plaisier, P.W., Berger, M.Y., van der Hul, R.L. *et al.* (1994) Unexpected difficulties in randomizing patients in a surgical trial: a prospective study comparing extracorporeal shock wave lithotripsy with open cholecystectomy. *World J Surg* **18**, 769–72

Pocock, S.J. (1984) *Clinical Trials; A Practical Approach.* Chichester: John Wiley

Russell, I. (1995) Evaluating new surgical procedures. *BMJ* **311**, 1243–4

Schulz, K.F., Chalmers, I., Haynes, R.J. and Altman, D.G. (1995) Empirical evidence of bias. Dimensions of methodological quality associated with estimates of treatment effects in controlled trials. *JAMA* **273**, 408–12

Sibbald, B. and Roland, M. (1998) Why are RCTs important? *BMJ* **316**, 201

Smithells, R., Sheppard, S., Schorah, C.J. *et al.* (1980) Possible prevention of neural-tube defects by periconceptional vitamin supplementation. *Lancet* **i**, 339–40

UK Collaborative ECMO Trial Group (1996) UK collaborative randomised trial of neonatal extracorporeal membrane oxygenation. *Lancet* **348**, 75–82

Wennberg, J.E. (1990) 'What is outcomes research?' in A.C. Gelijns (Ed.) *Medical Innovations at the Crossroads: Modern Methods of Clinical Investigation*, pp 33–46. Washington: National Academy Press

Zelen, M. (1979) A new design for randomized clinical trials. *New Engl J Med* **300**, 1242–5

## 11

Animal research

Fiona Broughton Pipkin

'... not in any way to be enterprised, nor taken in hand, unadvisedly, lightly or wantonly'

Solemnisation of Matrimony, The Book of Common Prayer.

The use of living animals in scientific procedures is highly contentious. In this chapter, I shall not consider work undertaken to comply with legislation, for example that relating to regulatory toxicology, but will concentrate entirely on biomedical research. Questions about ethics and scientific utility must be asked before any such work is undertaken. Absolutely central to the ethical dimension is the cost–benefit equation. This is because, as distinct from work involving human subjects, there can be no consent by an animal to participation in research. The individual animal will not benefit from any procedure, as may be the case in human clinical trials, nor will it be aware of its contribution to increasing the sum of knowledge. Its own species may benefit where findings have implications for veterinary medicine but, for our purposes, this is serendipity and not a primary objective. The animal thus bears all of the cost.

As with any research, before you start planning it you must be as sure as you can be that the answer to the question is worth having. This is the 'benefit' aspect of the cost–benefit equation. As in human-based research, it is a good idea to write down a formal list of benefits, rather than having a woolly idea at the back of your mind. Are you certain beyond reasonable doubt that the work has not been done before? If it has, have the results been conclusive? With on-line access to Medline and BIDS, there is no excuse for not knowing. It is essential for new researchers to talk through the concepts with a colleague experienced in this type of work.

Once you have decided that there are genuine benefits to be obtained and you think that your hypothesis can reasonably be tested in animals, stop and think again. Do you really have to use live animals? Increasing use is being made of isolated cells and cell or tissue cultures to answer questions at the molecular and genetic level. A good source of information about alternatives is FRAME[1] which, with the UFAW[2], has recently published a useful booklet

[1] Fund for the Replacement of Animals in Medical Experiments, Eastgate House, 34 Stoney Street, Nottingham NG1 1NB.
[2] Universities Federation for Animal Welfare, The Old School, Brewhouse Hill, Wheathampstead, Hertfordshire AL4 8AN.

on replacement models (FRAME and UFAW 1998). At the other end of the scale, the development of increasingly sophisticated techniques for measuring physiological variables non- or minimally invasively in man may mean that a question relating to integrated physiology can now be answered in the species in which you are primarily interested. Have you really investigated these possibilities?

If you cannot undertake the work in human volunteers, will data obtained from animals be of use in relation to man? Much is; some is not. For example, the unravelling of the story of lung surfactant and its vital role in the transition to extrauterine life was almost all carried out in the fetal and newborn lamb and rabbit. These data were directly applicable across species and have proved invaluable. The prenatal administration of glucocorticoids in the treatment of very prematurely delivered babies is a clear example of the value of curiosity-driven research generating hypotheses, tested in animals and resulting in the development of entirely novel therapeutic measures. Conversely, some aspects of placental physiology in the sheep differ markedly from our own.

If you conclude that you must use animals and that data so obtained will be relevant to your human patients, then consider what is the most suitable species to use. It may be possible to use an invertebrate species; our understanding of mammalian nerve conduction has been built on the giant axon of the squid. In considering the use of vertebrates, it is sometimes argued that the life of a rat or mouse is equivalent to that of a dog, cat or primate. This is not generally or instinctively felt to be appropriate in this context. Therefore, if you can use rats or mice, do so. On the other hand, if the question can only properly be answered using a higher species, then use that species. Remember that a careful choice of model should lead to more rapid advances in understanding and therefore keep the number of animals used to a minimum. The use of primates should be avoided if at all possible.

Where would the work be done? All experimental work involving the use of living animals in the United Kingdom comes under the Animals (Scientific Procedures) Act 1986, and may only be performed in places holding a Certificate of Designation (see below). Make contact with your university's animal house, talk to those who would be in day-to-day charge of the animals. Talk to the veterinary surgeon with responsibility for the animal house. Quite apart from any surgical and experimental skills which may be required, there will be questions of suitable anaesthetic techniques, postoperative care if recovery experiments are to be performed, the determination of clinical end-points mandating the humane killing of the animal, regardless of whether the experiment is complete or not, and the final euthanasia of the animal. The Laboratory Animals Science Association and UFAW publish a useful series of booklets entitled *Guidelines on the Care of Laboratory Animals and their Use for Scientific Purposes.*

Are your clinical commitments such that you can in fact 'ring-fence' the amount of time required for the work, which is likely to be more than you think? If you cannot unequivocally answer 'yes', then you should obtain funding for a co-worker, whose primary responsibility is the animal work. Attempting to squeeze experimental work into slots in a demanding clinical schedule all too often results in poorly conducted or unfinished studies and the consequent waste of animals' lives.

Experiments must be designed in association with a statistician to ensure not only that the minimum number of animals needed to test the hypothesis is used, but also that sufficient animals are used to test it properly. Poor science is unpublishable and unethical.

You should familiarise yourself at an early stage in planning your work with the concept of 'The three Rs' – reduction, refinement and replacement – and try to think it through in the context of that work. 'Refinement' in this context implies the introduction of methods which alleviate or minimise the pain, distress or other adverse effects which may be suffered by experimental animals, and/or enhance their general well-being. Quite apart from the priorities of the application of ethical and humane principles, it should always be remembered that a 'stressed' animal will not give physiologically useful data. The Boyd Group is a discussion forum which brings together individuals from responsible animal rights and welfare groups, practising scientists and ethicists, and sets up working groups to discuss particular topics in relation to the use of animals in biomedical research. They have recently published a useful article on current concepts of refinement in animal use (Boyd Group 1998).

The ethical review process

At this stage you will have done your detailed background reading, formulated your hypothesis, thought through the cost–benefit equation, investigated alternatives, chosen your species, decided where the work would be done and designed your experiment. You will have discussed the work with a variety of colleagues. You must now submit your work to your local Animal Care and Use Committee for approval.

It is an administrative requirement under the 1986 Act that '…an ethical review process be established and maintained at each establishment designated under the … Act.' Such review must be tailored to meet the needs of the establishment and the aims of the policy. The Animal Procedures Committee, which oversees the workings of the 1986 Act (see below) gave information about five possible models for establishment-based ethical review in its 1995 Report (Animal Procedures Committee 1996). Either the senior colleague who will be advising on the work, or the head technician in your animal house will be able to tell you what are the local arrangements for this committee. Such committees go by various names, but their function is to check that you have indeed gone through all the preliminaries with proper care and that the work is ethically acceptable within your community. Your next step is to acquire the authority under the 1986 Act to perform the work.

The Animals (Scientific Procedures) Act 1986

It is a criminal offence to perform any procedure on a living vertebrate animal (and some cephalopods) for purposes of research unless the programme of work is authorised by a Project Licence, issued by the Home Secretary, and the person undertaking the procedure is the holder of a Personal Licence. It does not matter how experienced a clinician you are, there are no exemptions. Everyone applying for a Personal Licence must undergo formal training through an accredited training scheme and be certified as having successfully done so. Consult the head technician in your animal house for details of local arrangements.

You must then fill out a detailed application form for a Personal Licence, for permission to undertake the procedures which you yourself will be performing. Once awarded, the Personal Licence authorises you to undertake only those procedures; if you subsequently discover that you need to use other procedures, further formal authorisation must be sought, and given, before they can be used. Personal Licences may only be used in conjunction with a Project Licence.

A Project Licence authorises a programme of work which requires the application of specified regulated procedures to animals of specified descriptions at a specified place or places. It is granted by the Home Secretary to the person who undertakes overall responsibility for the programme specified in that licence. If you are new to work with animals, it is strongly advised that you identify a senior colleague with relevant experience to advise you and collaborate with you. It may be appropriate and possible for you to work initially under their Project Licence although to do so will require an authorised modification of that project licence (see above).

Once written, the applications for Project and Personal Licences are sent to the Home Office for authorisation. This usually takes several months and no work may be undertaken until the licences have been awarded. Writing the applications for these licences and getting them can easily take four to six months.

Overseeing the workings of the Act in the university where you work will be an inspector from the Home Office. They will be a registered medical or veterinary practitioner, who makes both scheduled and unscheduled visits to the university. You should arrange to meet them as soon as you begin to consider doing work with living animals. They will be able to advise on administrative procedures for your applications and on such matters as potential local advisers and collaborators (see above). It is also helpful for the inspector to be forewarned of the area of work for which an application may be submitted, so that they can do any necessary background reading.

Work may only be carried out in a place designated as a scientific establishment by a Certificate issued by the Home Secretary. In academic life, the 'Certificate holder' is almost invariably a senior member of the university's administrative staff, such as the Registrar or Assistant Registrar. They are responsible for ensuring, through a clear management line, that all work undertaken under the Act is in accordance with it. You are responsible for ensuring that you understand this management line and comply with its requirements.

You are legally required to submit a return of all work performed under the Act in one year in the early spring of the following year. The legal requirements for note keeping are covered in the training course. Laboratory notebooks are, of course, extremely important scientifically and must also be available to the inspector on request at any time.

Informing the public

The UK has a long, honourable and worldwide reputation for the concern of its population for the well-being of animals, whether domesticated or wild. However, a large and increasing proportion of that population is now urban or suburban and only comes into direct contact with living animals under highly artificial circumstances. Its anthropomorphic perceptions of the animal kingdom frequently appear to be based on those of sentimentalising media and cartoon characters. In contrast, biomedical scientists are too often portrayed by the same media as ghouls, even though in their daily lives those exposed to these same media benefit from the eventual outcomes of animal research. An industry has grown up which attempts to convince schoolchildren that research using living animals is intrinsically and always unjustifiable. It receives generous funding from several 'animal welfare' charities. Debate should most certainly be stimulated on the topic, but it must be informed from both sides to be of any value.

No-one should undertake research using living animals unless they and their peers are convinced of the value of, and justification for, so doing. Once you have decided that such work is valuable and justified, and begun publishing so that the work is in the public domain, think about agreeing to take part in local debates, whether in a school or college, or on local radio or television. The Research Defence Society[3] will give expert help in preparing you for such a role; do make use of them. This gives you the opportunity to explain and justify why such work is necessary, to point out any direct implications of your work for clinical care and to describe the numerous levels of controls which have to be gone through before and during any such work. It is disgraceful that a few violent extremists should have terrorised some research workers to the point where they are unwilling to speak about their work publicly other than at scientific meetings. Such extremists have no place in an educated and thinking society.

[3] Research Defence Society, 58 Great Marlborough Street, London W1V 1DD.

References

Animal Procedures Committee (1996) *Report of the Animal Procedures Committee for 1995.* London: HMSO

Animals (Scientific Procedures) Act 1986. London: HMSO

Boyd Group (1998) Advancing refinement of laboratory animal use. *Lab Anim* **32**, 1-6

FRAME and UFAW (1998) *Selection and Use of Replacement Methods in Animal Experimentation.* (Obtainable from FRAME)

## 12

Fetal research

Nicholas M. Fisk

The problem

The sanctity of the fetal environment provides a formidable barrier to research endeavour. While the fetus lies, inaccessible, within the pregnant abdomen, it is also vulnerable to exogenous insults causing teratogenicity, miscarriage and prematurity. Mothers, understandably, regard their babies as 'precious' and ethical constraints preclude all but 'trivial risk' research. Whereas adult medicine advances apace due to modern technology, fetal medicine lags well behind, denied the progress in knowledge that would accrue from positron emission tomography, nuclear medicine, interventional radiology, metabolic challenge, cardiac catheterisation, direct drug therapy, invasive circulatory monitoring, chronic arterial or venous access and serial tissue biopsy.

The field

The modern subspecialty of fetal medicine owes its origins to two parallel developments, the advent of high resolution ultrasound and the access to the fetus provided by modern invasive procedures. In particular, fetal blood sampling allowed biochemical and haematological investigation as well as direct therapy by transfusion or injection. Despite considerable research activity using these tools over the last 10–15 years, many questions remain. In physiological terms, for instance, we do not understand what causes circulatory redistribution ('brain sparing') in response to hypoxaemia, while in clinical terms there has yet to be a randomised controlled trial (RCT) for any invasive fetal therapy.

Fetal medicine, however, is by no means limited to ultrasound and invasive procedures. A glance at the index of any of the mainstream journals in obstetrics and gynaecology reveals that around half of published articles deal with the fetus and/or placenta. The 'big three' problems in obstetric practice, preterm labour, growth restriction and pre-eclampsia, are arguably more fetal than maternal, their origins lying with impaired trophoblastic invasion, or altered signalling between the fetus and placenta/membranes. Miscarriage also is most commonly due to fetal causes, while the immunology of pregnancy, in particular the non-rejection of the fetoplacental allograft, remains a puzzle. Transplacental drug therapy provides two of the very few proven successful treatments in obstetrics: corticosteroids to enhance lung maturity, and periconceptual folate to prevent neural tube defects. Finally, the genetic revolution resulting from advances in molecular biology, together with the human genome project, will have a major impact, not just in prenatal diagnosis and disease susceptibility, but also in developing better therapies, particularly drugs. Although gene therapy has so far been disappointing, with little application *in utero*, the theoretical advantages of intrauterine stem cell transplantation may, in the future, render this the preferred approach for transfection of autologous cells to cure paediatric and adult disease.

Fetal ethics

Ethics, law and public moral sensitivity vary widely from country to country. In those countries where termination is proscribed, some types of fetal research may be problematic, not only those involving fetal tissues but also those involving invasive procedures, the predominant indication for which is fetal karyotyping. On the other hand there is, instead, opportunity for other forms of research not possible elsewhere, such as the prediction of neurological outcome in fetuses with open spina bifida.

This section is necessarily parochial, based on UK practice, but its principles are applicable to many other jurisdictions. Fetal research in the UK is governed by the 1989 report of the Polkinghorne Committee entitled *Code of Practice on the Use of Fetuses and Fetal Material in Research and Treatment*, the chief recommendations of which were accepted by the Government and now determine ethics committee approval.

Live fetuses

Under UK law, the fetus is not considered a person at any gestation and has no independent legal rights before birth. Beneficence-based ethics holds that, in continuing pregnancies, the mother bestows moral status on her fetus and, thus, the obligation to do good rather than harm. It has been argued that the fetus acquires independent moral status (i.e. independent of maternal intent) after viability, although this appears overly simplistic in countries such as the UK where the mother can elect to undergo late termination of a fetus at substantial risk of severe handicap (Chervenak and McCullough 1997).

The Polkinghorne report recommended that research on living fetuses should be treated on principles broadly comparable to those applicable to children and adults, which preclude intervention above minimal risk. More stringent ethical principles pertaining to research on children are considered to apply particularly to the fetus. These preclude procedures of anything more than 'trivial risk', equated to that of a transatlantic flight, except where the balance of benefit is to the fetus.

Dead fetuses

Most fetal tissue for research is derived from terminated fetuses. Tissue can be used after spontaneous fetal demise, but there are real difficulties. These relate to not only the normality and representative nature of the specimens, such as after first trimester miscarriage, but also to post-mortem changes in the interval from demise until delivery, the latter precluding all gene expression studies and in many cases cytogenetic, immuno-cytochemical and histological investigation.

The guiding ethical principle of the Polkinghorne report is that the decisions and actions relating to the abortion process should be separated from the decisions and actions relating to use of the material. There are two main restrictions.

First, Section 3.4 states that 'the mother should not be informed of the specific use which may be made of fetal tissue, or whether it is to be used at all'. In my own institution, patients are asked to sign a generic consent form:

> *I ... agree that the fetal tissues taken at the time of termination of pregnancy may be used for teaching, research or therapy. I understand that the use of this tissue will be strictly controlled according to official guidelines and restricted to uses for which fetal tissue is necessary for medical benefit. I understand that I will not be identified as the source of the fetal tissues if they are used for these purposes.*

This embargo on informed consent may create difficulties where maternal and paternal samples are required, such as for genetic testing or infection screening. There are also studies where the mother needs to consent to additional research procedures, such as transabdominal needling of the extra-embryonic coelom or yolk sac. Such protocols are best examined individually by ethics committees to see to what extent they comply with the Polkinghorne guidelines.

Secondly, Section 3.5 recommends that 'those involved in the process of abortion, and responsible for the clinical care of the mother should not knowingly be involved in research on the fetus or fetal tissue'. To facilitate this separation, the Government set up the MRC Fetal Tissue Bank in 1995, based at Hammersmith Hospital (Department of Health 1995). Research protocols in which the integrity of the specimen would be jeopardised by the use of frozen or only relatively fresh tissue from the bank can still be accommodated provided the above principles are honoured. The report acknowledges ethically acceptable exceptions to this degree of separation, principally in the investigation of fetal demise.

Other fetally derived tissues

The contents of the uterus other than the fetus (membranes, amniotic fluid and placenta) may be used under the Code, providing the mother consents to any additional screening tests and is not under financial inducement. Usage, however, is not subject to the restrictions under Section 3 above, nor the requirement to obtain ethics committee approval. Traditionally, ethical approval has not been considered necessary for research on tissues that would otherwise be discarded. However, ethical approval is now advisable, due to the increasingly stringent requirements of many journals, a greater parental sense of ownership of their placenta and increasing general standards of patient consent.

Clinical research

Like obstetrics in general, fetal research is beset by the problem of numbers: pathological fetuses and pregnancies are rare amid an overwhelming background of normal pregnancies. The importance of paying attention to the power in any study design is emphasised elsewhere in this book; essentially to achieve sufficient power, research on fetal abnormalities or survival needs either to be conducted on high risk groups and referral populations, or to be multi-centre.

Epidemiology and audit

Audit of practice in individual centres provided much of the early insights into fetal medicine. With computerised databases and increasing caseload in referral centres, reasonable data now exist on the outcome of prenatally diagnosed abnormalities and the frequency of aneuploidy in association with various ultrasonic markers. The latter have largely been univariate analyses with single markers and researchers have only recently begun to derive multi-parameter aneuploidy risks. Audit of fetal outcome after various anomalies or invasive procedures in individual centres does have a local role in education and maintenance of standards, but it is unlikely to contribute to the literature unless it is applied over several centres or based on large numbers over many years.

Publications from referral centres are necessarily biased by the selected nature of their referral population. Epidemiological studies yield more representative information based on regional or national data. Examples include regional congenital malformation registries, data from the Office of National Statistics on Down syndrome and termination for fetal abnormality (Filatki 1997) and surveillance data on toxoplasmosis reported to the British Paediatric Association (Lynn and Hall 1992). The analysis of such data is relatively straightforward; the difficulty lies in instituting a prospective system of uniform reporting with complete ascertainment.

Observational research

This comprises the bulk of published research to date in fetal medicine. It typically involves ultrasound and/or Doppler observations, either longitudinally, to determine pregnancy changes and outcome, or cross-sectional comparisons of normal with abnormal fetuses. The popularity of this type of research stems from its ethical simplicity and the ready availability of clinical material. The longer the subspecialty exists, however, the less original this type of research becomes. Notwithstanding this, observational studies will continue to generate novel data due to advances in imaging, such as:

- 3D scanning

- colour energy and harmonic ultrasound
- ultra-fast magnetic resonance imaging
- contrast agents
- advances in Doppler methods, allowing the study of increasingly smaller fetal vessels, such as the coronary and adrenal arteries.

Special consideration needs to be given to comparing groups of fetuses at different gestations. Analysis of covariance can be used to control for gestational age in studies of relatively small numbers, but the preferred technique involves expressing variables in gestational independent z-scores or standard deviations. The construction of a normal or reference range across gestation is complex, requiring attention not only to sufficient numbers but also to the normality of distribution across gestation (Royston 1991). As a general rule, 20 patients are required for construction of a longitudinal reference range, and 100–200 for a cross-sectional one.

Before reporting abnormal findings, one must be confident of what is normal and here a sound grounding in fetal physiology is advantageous. Much research in this area has been done by those whose predominant interest lies, not in fetal medicine, but in ultrasound, often more generally applied to obstetrics and gynaecology. This has perpetuated several misconceptions, such as in relation to the predictive value of fetal breathing movements which, by definition, are episodic in nature and change markedly in pattern with fetal maturation.

A further difficulty arises when evaluating tests of fetal well-being, if these are disclosed to clinicians. A useless test to predict perinatal survival may appear beneficial in such trials, if the treatment instituted is of value, i.e. delivery. Alternatively, a very useful test will not appear so if the intervention is useless. Once non-disclosure trials have confirmed associations with adverse outcome, the clinical utility of disclosing such information to clinicians should be evaluated in randomised trials. A good example of this is the development of umbilical artery Doppler monitoring in high risk pregnancies, the only diagnostic test shown in RCTs to reduce perinatal mortality (Alfirevic and Neilson 1995).

Invasive procedures

The access to the fetus provided by invasive procedures, in particular fetal blood sampling, led to a plethora of important observational studies in the late 1980s, which established baseline biochemical, haematological, immunological and endocrinological parameters. This procedure has been in relative decline in the 1990s due to more rapid non-blood karyotyping techniques, PCR-based diagnosis in amniotic fluid, better risk estimation from ultrasound findings and Doppler to predict fetal well-being (Fisk and Bower 1993). Accordingly, many units have set up banks of small additional aliquots of fetal blood and other fluids collected routinely with ethical approval at clinically indicated fetal blood and other sampling procedures. A typical design has been to compare parameters in groups of pathological fetuses with those of control fetuses, usually those undergoing genetic testing which proves normal. Much of the interesting research has been done, although the discovery of new enzymes, hormones and cytokines, as well as new conditions (for instance the hereditary thromobophilias) will see this remain a useful research tool.

Because fetal blood sampling carries more than a trivial risk to the fetus, it seems unlikely that ethics committees would approve fetal blood sampling for non-therapeutic research purposes alone. Notwithstanding this, a couple of groups have used fetal blood sampling to investigate preterm labour, with one American group arguing that this practice is acceptable providing the mother is fully informed (Berry *et al.* 1997). On the other hand, therapeutic research involving risky invasive procedures should prove acceptable to ethics committees, providing there is, on balance, a prospect of more good than harm to the fetal patient.

There are special difficulties with evaluating invasive procedures. Ideally, these should be compared in RCTs with control groups not undergoing an invasive procedure. This creates understandable difficulty with recruitment. For diagnostic procedures, patients are reluctant to accept a chance of randomisation to no diagnostic test, while for invasive therapies such as vesico-amniotic shunting, many parents are keen to do everything possible for their fetus, even if the proposed treatment is experimental. It is worth remembering that there has been only one trial with randomisation to an invasive versus no procedure (Tabor *et al.* 1986). It is almost impossible to envisage women with high-order multiple pregnancies consenting to a randomised trial of multi-fetal pregnancy reduction versus conservative management.

Most of the diagnostic procedures have thus been evaluated against other invasive procedures, i.e. amniocentesis versus chorion villus sampling (CVS), transabdominal versus transcervical CVS. Even here, recruitment difficulties can limit the power of an RCT where patients are allowed to choose their preferred procedure outside randomisation. One way around this is to confine offers of a new procedure within the context of an RCT, although to be effective this may require a national approach such as happened in Canada with the introduction of CVS.

No matter how attractive, new procedures must always undergo evaluation, because of the possibility that they may be deleterious. An example is the theoretically attractive procedure of early amniocentesis, now shown in several randomised trials to cause talipes and to have a higher miscarriage rate than CVS (Wilson *et al.* 1998). A further difficulty is deciding at what time in its development a procedure should be subjected to an RCT; too early and the results may mislead due to inexperience with the technique, too late and there may be recruitment difficulties.

Many of the newer procedures have very infrequent indications, such as fetal endoscopy and vascular ablation techniques. For these, evaluation by case series, comparison with historical and then non-randomised controls seems initially acceptable. Nevertheless, there has still been no assessment of efficacy for some rare procedures in use for over ten years, such as vesico-amniotic shunting. Pooling multi-centre experience is one way around this, as is Bayesian analysis of prior belief adjustment, whereby results are expressed in terms of the percentage chance that a treatment is beneficial (i.e. 90%) rather than rejected as of no benefit when the *P* value falls short of conventional significance (i.e. $P = 0.25$). RCTs remain the ideal although, as Lilford points out, the numbers are against them, with a population of 12 million pregnancies required for adequate power for a trial of shunting fetuses with pleural effusions (Lilford *et al.* 1995).

Drugs

Fetal medicine as a branch of medical practice uses surprisingly few drugs. Only peri-conceptual folate to prevent spina bifida and corticosteroids to mature fetal lungs are of proven benefit. Any role for others, such as immunoglobulin therapy in alloimmune disease or prophylactic low-dose aspirin to prevent vascular complications, remains controversial. Further drugs may even harm the fetus, such as long-term use of the tocolytic, indomethacin. The mode of drug delivery may also prove problematic, as illustrated by anti-arrhythmic drugs which on one hand cross the placenta poorly, especially in the presence of hydrops, while on the other hand their direct administration to the fetus necessitates excessively frequent intrauterine procedures. Drug carrier systems, such as liposomes, may be used in future to retard or facilitate transplacental drug passage (Bajoria *et al.* 1997).

Although the risk of teratogenicity (remember thalidomide and stilboestrol) provides powerful disincentives to experimentation in this area, such risks are largely confined to the first trimester. Because the Medicines Licensing Act 1968 permits individual doctors to prescribe drugs for unlicensed use on their own responsibility, drug companies with product licences for non-obstetric drugs with obstetric applications are understandably reluctant to do research in this area. This explains why few drugs are licensed for use in pregnancy, other than those with a pregnancy-only application, such as tocolytics and uterotonics. Indeed, corticosteroids to enhance lung maturity remain unlicensed for this purpose (Fisk and Shennan 1993). This retards research in obstetric therapeutics, by preventing drug company funding.

Anyone proposing a trial involving an unlicensed drug or a licensed drug not licensed for that particular purpose in pregnancy (i.e. almost all drugs), will require, in addition to ethical approval, a Doctors' Exemption Certificate from the Medicine's Licensing Authority.

Laboratory research

Animal

The advantages are two-fold. First, there are fewer ethical constraints, which means that invasive, longitudinal and terminal studies with immediate access to pathological tissue are feasible. Secondly, robust design controls for the numerous variables which beleaguer clinical studies, so much so that study numbers of six in each group (intervention and control) often yield significant results. The catheterised fetal sheep has proved a popular model, although chronic experiments remain a challenge, despite the relative inertia of the ovine uterus. Because their placentation is different to that in humans, being epitheliochorial and cotyledonary, non-human primate models with their single disc haemochorial placentae are preferred; their use in all but a few centres, however, has been precluded by high cost, greater ethical consideration and extremely stringent licensing requirements. Smaller animals are used for drug studies and increasingly 'knock out' mice lacking a certain gene provide useful insights into embryology and teratogenesis. See Chapter 11 for a full discussion of research using animals.

Trophoblast and placenta

The dually-perfused isolated placental lobule which aims to mimic the feto-placental and utero-placental circulations *in vitro* is commonly used to study placental transfer under experimental conditions. It remains viable for up to a few hours, sufficient for study of bi-directional transport and equilibration. Concerns about the non-physiological nature of such perfusion can be addressed in part by serial monitoring of perfusion, flow and pressure, pH and acid-base status, although even under optimal conditions these still differ from those found *in vivo*. The disadvantages of this model are that technical considerations largely limit it to study of the full-term (normal) placenta, not those complicated by growth restriction, pre-eclampsia, infection or hydrops earlier in pregnancy. An alternative is to study trans-placental transfer of drugs at fetal blood sampling, although this precludes use of radio labels and is limited to pregnancies with a clinical indication both for drug administration and fetal blood sampling.

Microvillus membrane preparations of syncytiotrophoblast are used to study the mechanism of transfer across the placenta (i.e. endocytosis, para-cellular channels etc.). Cell lines of trophoblast can be used to study cell signalling and decidual interactions, although there remains concern about the maintenance of a cell's native characteristics following the immortalisation process. Finally, placental bed biopsies are used in pathological pregnancies in an attempt to understand the cellular events mediating impaired trophoblast invasion. A major limitation is that these are obtained months after the primary and secondary waves of trophoblast invasion and, as such, represent only the burnt out embers of the disease process.

Molecular biology

Molecular genetic techniques are no longer the province of molecular biologists and, instead, are used in virtually all laboratory-based research as tools to investigate integrated physiology and disease processes. Although much work has been done on conventional DNA testing by PCR for inherited disease in the field of prenatal diagnosis, detecting mRNA using reverse transcriptase PCR and Northern blotting is integral to determining the expression and regulation of proteins and enzymes in any reproductive tissue, such as hormones and cytokines regulating the onset of labour in membranes and myometrium. With the human genome mapping project due to be complete within the next two years, an increasing number of disease susceptibility genes will be cloned. An example may be that for obstetric cholestasis, following which a reverse genetic approach could be used, as it was for cystic fibrosis, to determine the protein basis of this disorder and, ideally, to develop rational drug therapies. It is also likely that more genes influencing multifactorial conditions will be identified; examples so far include the wild type methyltetrahydrofolate reductase variant in mothers at risk of neural tube defects and glucokinase variants in growth restriction.

Advances in molecular methods should allow prenatal karyotyping on amniotic fluid without need for culture, either by multiprobe fluorescent *in situ* hybridisation or by DNA quantitation of short tandem repeats situated near each centromere. Rare event techniques should eventually see non-invasive prenatal diagnosis in fetal cells in the maternal circulation become a reality. Increasingly, intrauterine events are being implicated in later onset disease. Although the Barker hypothesis is well known, studies of feto-maternal cell trafficking have more recently implicated persistent fetal cells in the maternal blood stream in the aetiology of scleroderma and possibly exposure to non-inherited maternal antigens *in utero* in the aetiology of auto-immune diseases.

Advice

Remember, research is not difficult, but it is a learnt exercise; therefore, choosing a sympathetic and productive supervisor is a sensible first step. In selecting a hypothesis to test, first pick something achievable within local conditions and facilities. Although it is important to be inspired by your own question, a more pragmatic approach is to look around at the strengths, expertise and clinical material available in your own centre, as these will determine both the feasibility and originality of your project. Laboratory research is more controlled and requires a greater time commitment, while clinical research is subject to the vagaries of patient numbers, consent and clinical variation. This may explain why there have been few peer review research grants awarded in clinical fetal medicine research.

Despite the ethical and accessibility problems, fetal research remains a field with many challenging clinical and scientific questions (Fisk 1998). The stakes are high, not just because fetal disease is associated with high perinatal morbidity and mortality, but because the intrauterine environment has longer term affects on health. These constraints on fetal research should be seen as challenges.

References

Alfirevic, Z. and Neilson, J. (1995) Doppler ultrasonography in high-risk pregnancies: systematic review with meta-analysis. *Am J Obstet Gynecol* **172**, 1379–87

Bajoria, R., Fisk, N.M. and Contractor, S.F. (1997) Liposomal thyroxine: a non-invasive model for transplacental fetal therapy. *J Clin Endocrinol Metab* **82**, 3271–7

Berry, S., Romero, R., Ghezzi, F. *et al.* (1997) Risks and ethical issues of the use of diagnostic cordocentesis in the evaluation of fetuses with preterm labor. Proceedings of the 17th Annual Meeting of the Society of Perinatal Obstetricians, Anaheim, California. *Am J Obstet Gynecol* **176**, S20

Chervenak, F. and McCullough, L. (1997) 'Ethics of fetal therapy' in: N.M. Fisk and K.J. Moise Jr (Eds) *Fetal Therapy: Invasive and Transplacental,* pp. 345–56. Cambridge: Cambridge University Press

Committee to Review the Guidance on the Research Use of Fetuses and Fetal Material (1989) *Report of the Committee to Review the Guidance on the Research Use of Fetuses and Fetal Material, Sections 1–7* (Cm 762). London: HMSO

Department of Health (1995) *Guidance on the Use of Fetal Tissue for Research, Diagnosis and Therapy.* London: Department of Health

Filakti, H. (1997) Trends in abortion 1990–1995. *Popul Trends* **87**, 11–19

Fisk, N.M. (1998) Maternal-fetal medicine and prenatal diagnosis – editorial comment. *Curr Opin Obstet Gynecol* **10**, 81–4

Fisk, N.M. and Bower, S. (1993) Fetal blood sampling in retreat. *BMJ* **307**, 143–4

Fisk, N.M. and Shennan, A.H. (1993) Litigation and prescribing drugs for unlicensed indications. *Lancet* **341**, 1218

Lilford, R.J., Thornton, J.G. and Braunholtz, D. (1995) Clinical trials and rare diseases: a way out of a conundrum. *BMJ* **311**, 1621–5

Lynn, R. and Hall, S.M. (1992) The British Paediatric Surveillance Unit: activities and developments in 1990 and 1991. *Commun Dis Rep (CDR) Rev* **2**, R145–8

Royston, P. (1991) Constructing time-specific reference ranges. *Stat Med* **10**, 675–90

Tabor, A., Philip, J., Madsen, M. *et al.* (1986) Randomised controlled trial of genetic amniocentesis in 4606 low-risk women. *Lancet* **1**, 1287–93

Wilson, R.D., Johnson, J.M., Dansereau, J. *et al.* (1998) Randomised trial to assess safety and fetal outcome of early and midtrimester amniocentesis. *Lancet* **351**, 242–7

13

Laboratory research and quality control

D. Stephen Charnock-Jones

Many of the principles underlying good quality laboratory research are also of fundamental importance to non-laboratory-based research. However, when carrying out laboratory-based work one can readily get distracted by the technology and lose sight of the principles which underlie high quality research. This is particularly true in fields which make use of modern cellular and molecular techniques where many complex steps are necessary before one actually performs the true experiment.

An essential first step in all research is the formulation of the hypothesis to be tested. Ideally, this should be clear, simple and short. Once this has been formulated, the design of the experiments to test this hypothesis should be relatively straightforward. At this point, it is essential to ensure that the experiments proposed do indeed test the hypothesis. While designing these experiments, it is essential to identify what controls will be needed. Some of these will be controls required for the actual hypothesis testing, but in laboratory-based studies there may well be additional controls necessary to ensure that the assay or reagents are working as expected. Specific examples of such studies are given later.

Modern biomedical research has developed rapidly in the last 20 years and continues to do so at an increasing pace. The use of cellular and molecular techniques to understand the biochemical and genetic basis of health and disease has radically altered our understanding of physiology. However, to perform such experiments, complex biochemical and/or genetic techniques are required which use many specialised reagents. It is, therefore, of fundamental importance that the reagents, be they antibodies, probes or oligonucleotides, are well characterised and their performance verified during the course of an experimental procedure.

Are you sure you are measuring what you think you are measuring?

In this context, it is of paramount importance that all probes and antibodies are validated for the use to which they are to be put. DNA probes (including oligonucleotides) should be sequenced and checked for specificity. This is particularly important for DNA probes which may contain repeated sequences or are derived from regions of genes which may be conserved. The latter can include control regions of promoters but also functional domains of coding sequences. Derivation of a shorter DNA probe may well actually improve specificity although it can reduce sensitivity.

Validation of antibody performance is more problematical than that for DNA probes and this is particularly true when antibodies are to be used for immunohistochemistry. Ideally, the performance of an antibody used for immunlocalisation should be compared with localisation studies using alternative techniques, for example, radioligand binding or *in situ* hybridisation. However, this is frequently impossible and therefore one may resort to Western blotting to demonstrate that the antibody indeed recognises an antigen of the expected molecular weight.

While a successful Western blot gives considerable reassurance of the specificity of an antibody, failure to achieve success using this particular technique does not necessarily mean that immunostaining in tissue sections is invalid. For example, if the immunolocalisation is confined to a very rare population of cells in the section, then the antigen may be undetectable when tissue is homogenised and analysed by Western blotting. In any event, the appropriate controls must be performed when carrying out immunohistology. These include for monoclonal antibodies, use of an isotope-matched control and for polyclonal antibodies, the use of non-immune serum of the same species (if possible pre-immune serum from the same animal). Where the antibody has been raised against a synthetic peptide pre-absorption of the antisera with an excess of the peptide should be performed. However, it is possible still to have spurious staining which appears to be specific since it can be obliterated by such pre-absorption. This is thought to occur because of shared but unidentified epitopes in the peptide which are also common to several antigens present within the tissue. When describing the results of immunohistochemistry, the experimenter should take care in the description of the result. Specifically, 'antigen-like immunoreactivity' is what has been localised, not the protein, and neither of these equates in any way to a demonstration of gene expression.

Antibodies are also commonly used in radio immunoassays and enzyme linked immunosorbant assays (RIA and ELISA); again, using these quantitative assays it is essential that the antibody and antigen labelling are both validated. Antibody specificity is of paramount importance when measuring levels of closely related analytes (for example, related steroid hormones or prostanoids). When such relatively small organic compounds are being assayed the radiolabel is usually incorporated directly into the antigen and does not alter its chemical structure. However, it is common when measuring peptides, polypeptides and proteins for the radiolabel (or indeed other label) to be chemically attached to the antigen. In such cases, it is essential to demonstrate that the iodination or biotinylation (for example) of the peptide or protein has not resulted in an alteration in antigen immunoreactivity. In addition, it is essential to demonstrate that dilutions of the sample are parallel to dilutions of the standard curve and that 'spike and recover' experiments give reproducible and consistent recoveries. Finally, it is important that internal controls should be included in every assay to allow ongoing determination of the inter- and intra-assay coefficients of variation.

These points are clearly of great importance to anyone wishing to develop an immunoassay; however, users of commercial assays should be aware that even these assays need to be validated and while the purchaser may expect that the supplier of the assay will have carried out such validation the demonstration of parallelism between the specific samples being used by the researcher and the standard curve is a valuable test to run.

The two examples of Northern blotting and the polymerase chain reaction given below illustrate the steps that need to be taken to ensure that a valid experiment is performed using these techniques. Without validation of the assays, hypothesis testing becomes impossible.

Example 1: Northern blotting

This is a widely used and straightforward technique which identifies and possibly quantifies the messenger RNA (mRNA) encoding a specific gene product within a population of RNA isolated from either cells or tissue. However, the apparent simplicity belies the underlying factors every researcher must consider. The points to be considered are:

- Sample selection: this will depend on the hypothesis to be tested but should include appropriate controls, for example, treated versus untreated cells or tissues; RNA from affected or unaffected individuals (attention needs to be paid as to how these are identified, how rigorous this selection is and how many replicates of each sample are to be analysed).

- The RNA samples to be run on the gel should all be prepared in the same way, the amount of RNA should be quantified and its integrity demonstrated.

- Appropriate molecular weight markers need to be run on the gel, as do additional samples which demonstrate the specificity of the probe to be used subsequently (a positive and a negative control).

- The gel needs to be run and the RNA transferred to the blotting membrane. Since the RNA can be degraded during each of these processes, some sort of staining of the membrane should be performed on the membrane to demonstrate that RNA has successfully been transferred and is still intact.

- The probe which is to be used in the hybridisation study should be characterised (by DNA sequencing). The purity and concentration of the probe need to be determined prior to labelling and the efficiency of labelling also needs to be determined.

- The hybridisation and washing conditions to be used may need to be refined by preliminary experimentation. However, this is only possible once a suitable positive control and probe have been identified.

- After autoradiography, the probe should be removed and the filter re-probed with an additional probe which hybridises to a housekeeping gene. This serves as a control to demonstrate that the loading of the gel and transfer to the membrane was even and that there was hybridisable RNA present in every lane.

While Northern blotting is one of the simplest techniques used in modern molecular biology, from this list it is obvious that there are numerous steps which can go wrong and which need to be validated during the course of the experiment. While most of them are relatively simple, they should not be overlooked.

Example 2: polymerase chain reaction

The polymerase chain reaction (PCR) is the workhorse of modern molecular biology and is based on the *in vitro* amplification of double-stranded DNA using a thermostable DNA polymerase. Again, its simplicity belies the underlying complexity and the pitfalls which await the unwary. The key questions to be considered by the researcher in performing these PCR reactions can be summed up in two questions.

- Did the reaction work?
- Was there PCR template present?

Thus, when carrying out such reactions, it is essential to include controls to demonstrate that the primers, enzyme and buffer are all functioning and that the template added (cDNA or genomic DNA) can be successfully amplified using alternative primers. An additional control which is absolutely essential for PCR reactions is the 'no-template control'. This demonstrates that there was no contamination of any of the reagents with a small amount of template which would lead to a false positive result. The importance of this negative control cannot be emphasised enough since, due to the extreme sensitivity of the PCR reaction, very small amounts of contamination can very easily lead to false positive results.

An example where all these considerations have been taken into account is shown in Figure 13.1. From this, it can be seen that all the controls described above are included. This specific experiment set out to determine whether acidic FGF and basic FGF were expressed in the two endometrial carcinoma cell lines HEC1–A and HEC1–B. Thus, the integrity of the RNA and the PCR ability of the cDNA was tested by amplifying cDNA from these two cell lines and also from normal proliferative phase endometrium with primers specifically for VEGF. These samples are shown in lanes 2, 3 and 4. Lane 5 contains a negative control with no template, showing that the VEGF PCR reaction was not contaminated. Lanes 6 and 7 demonstrate that the PCR reaction designed to amplify acidic and basic FGF cDNA also worked when using cDNA from proliferative phase endometrium. The negative controls demon-

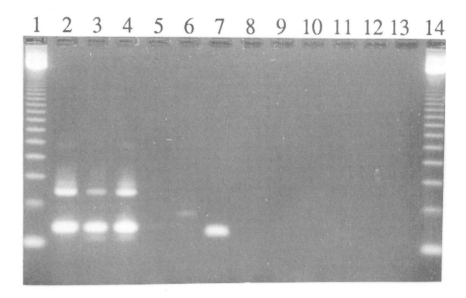

Figure 13.1 Agarose gel showing PCR products from the amplification of cDNA from the proliferative endometrium (lanes 2, 6 and 7), HEC1–A (lanes 3, 8 and 9), HEC1–B cell line (lanes 4, 10 and 11) and control (no template) (lanes 5, 12 and 13), with nested primers specific to VEGF (lanes 2, 3, 4 and 5), acidic FGF (lanes 6, 8, 10 and 12) and basic FGF (lanes 7, 9, 11 and 13). Lanes 1 and 14 are molecular weight markers (123bp ladder, BRL). Reproduced from Charnock-Jones *et al.* (1993) with permission

strating absence of contamination for the acidic and basic FGF PCR reactions are in lanes 12 and 13. The actual experimental lanes are lanes 8, 9, 10 and 11, in which cDNA from the two cell lines is amplified with primers specific for acidic or basic FGF. As can be seen, no PCR product is produced by these reactions. However, the other lanes on the gel demonstrate that the PCR reactions for acidic and basic FGF worked and that there was indeed intact cDNA present in the samples derived from the two cell lines in question. Thus, one can reliably conclude that acidic and basic FGF mRNA were either absent or below the level of sensitivity in this assay in the two endometrial carcinoma cell lines HEC1–A and HEC1–B.

Having formulated the hypothesis, designed rational experiments and carried them out using all the controls necessary both to validate the assays used and also as required by the hypothesis, one is left with the interpretation. A temptation at this point is to over-interpret the data and this should be resisted. For example, a common failing is to suggest that immunohistochemical localisation of an antigen means that there is local expression of the protein of interest. This is not the case. Strictly speaking, immunohistochemical localisation shows that there is an antigen-like immunoreactivity.

Conclusion

Thus, the essentials for good quality laboratory research can be summed up as follows:

* Have a good clear simple hypothesis.
* Design relevant experiments which test this.
* Perform experiments as designed, with the appropriate controls as required for the hypothesis and assay validation.
* Interpret cautiously.

Reference

Charnock-Jones, D.S., Sharkey, A.M., Rajput-Williams, J. *et al.* (1993) Identification and localization of alternately spliced mRNAs for vascular endothelial growth factor in human uterus and estrogen regulation in endometrial carcinoma cell lines. *Biol Reprod* **48**, 1120–8

## 14

Data management

Kirstie McKenzie-McHarg
and Sarah Ayers

In research, there is *nothing* more important than the quality of the data. This chapter will detail the issues that must be considered when you are planning and undertaking your research project. Once the research question has been formulated, the appropriate study design selected, the protocol written, funding obtained and ethics approval granted, answering the research question depends entirely on the data. Regardless of the size of your project, obtaining a complete and accurate data set should be your highest priority. Without valid, accurate, accessible and verifiable data you cannot obtain a reliable result in which people will have faith. Therefore, putting efficient data management systems into place early is crucial. Good data management is easy – it just requires a little thought, preferably before data collection begins.

Data management systems will necessarily vary immensely depending on your research design. You may be conducting a laboratory-based study, with all data being collected, collated and analysed by one person. At the more complex end, you may be running a large, multi-centre randomised controlled trial, involving hundreds of centres and thousands of subjects. In this chapter, we have assumed the most complex situation and will leave it to you to extract the information that best fits your needs.

What are the data? The data comprise every single item of information you collect for your study. Unfortunately, it is very easy to set up a study, collect the data and then discover that you have not recorded the information that will allow you to answer the research question in which you are interested. Therefore, it is crucial that you think about your final questions and what data you will need to answer these questions. It is also important that you do not collect redundant data – data that you will not use to answer any of the research questions in which you have an interest. Collecting redundant data wastes your time and the time of any other people involved in collecting them.

In multi-centre trials, there are sometimes 'dummy tables' to help you decide what data to collect. These should comprise the final data tables (blank, of course) which, as far as possible, will be used to produce the study results as defined in the protocol. However, for all studies, it is certainly worth spending some time considering the data you will need to collect in order to answer your research questions carefully and the forms that you will use to record the data you collect. Even in the case of a small, laboratory-based study, it is always worth producing a form for data collection. This ensures that your procedure is standardised and items are not missed. It makes checking your data easier and provides a record that will exist after the study is completed.

It is a good idea to ask people unconnected with the project to look at the forms or to try completing them in order to look for ambiguities and other problems which may not be apparent to the person designing the form. If at all possible, the forms should be piloted among the people who are going to be completing them in the final study. Once you have tested and verified the data form, the project can begin.

The issues involved in managing the data are numerous and each requires some preparation:

- complying with the Data Protection Act
- dealing with data on a day-to-day basis
- following-up missing data
- coding
- distinguishing missing data from data indicated as unknown (this is an important question which is often ignored)
- staff
- preparing for analysis
- deciding whether your data will be collected electronically or in paper format and crucially
- deciding how the data will be stored and backed-up.

The Data Protection Act

The Data Protection Act states that every effort must be made to maintain confidentiality of personal data held on a computer or stored in locked filing cabinets. Simultaneously, the system you devise needs to be workable, allowing authorised people easy access to data when needed, while preventing unauthorised access. This implies that all paperwork containing confidential or identifiable information should be locked away at all times, with restricted access to it, as well as restricted access to any data held on a computer. The Act also suggests that names and addresses should be stored separately from main outcome data so that non-project staff cannot link them together. This applies to both electronic and paper data.

Dealing with data on a day-to-day basis

This is where the type of research study you are conducting could have an enormous impact on the work you need to do in order to deal with your data efficiently. Again, we have assumed the most complex situation and a number of these points will not apply if you are collecting all the data yourself. However, many of the points are true regardless of the size of your project.

One of the first things you need to do is to develop a procedure for dealing with data forms when they begin returning to the study office. We recommend that you make this procedure a high priority on your list of tasks. You might want to consider something along the following lines:

- Data forms should be date-stamped on arrival, checked for completeness and 'checked in' whereby the arrival of the form is recorded, either electronically or on paper.
- If omissions or incomplete forms are discovered at this first check, you should return a photocopy of the data form, highlighting the omission/error to the study centre along with a covering letter. The original data form should *never* be returned to the person who filled it in asking them to resolve a query (you might never see it again).
- Once a form is complete, it should be filed in a manner that means you can find it again easily – most studies allocate a unique number to each subject and file paperwork consecutively by these subject numbers.

Following-up missing data

In the search for a complete and accurate data set, the following-up of missing data is one of the most crucial elements. This could take one of several forms.

In the first case, you may be awaiting data from an individual or an organisation (such as a hospital laboratory, hospital ward, GP clinic or NHS trust) that has not yet returned a questionnaire/data collection form. In the first instance, a system of automatic reminders should be instigated. The specifics of your project will play some part in helping you to decide how many postal reminders will be appropriate before you begin telephoning. If you are collecting information from a mother whose baby has died recently, it is unlikely that you would wish to contact her too often; however, if it is a case of determining a patient's blood pressure at a given moment from hospital case notes, you may need to contact the hospital frequently in order to obtain the information you need.

A second case could be where a questionnaire or form has been returned to you, but is incomplete in some detail. As you should not be collecting unimportant information, you should make every effort to pursue the missing data. As stated earlier, you should never send a form out of the data office once received – the chances are high that you will never receive it again. Instead, you should copy the original and send the copy, with missing information highlighted, to the person responsible for completing the form, together with a letter asking them to supply the missing information. A flowchart of this process is included in Figure 14.1.

Coding

Once you have all the data you can possibly obtain in your possession, coding may need to take place. Some forms of qualitative research (see Chapter 15 on analysis for a description of qualitative and quantitative research), especially those demanding content analysis, may transcribe conversations or

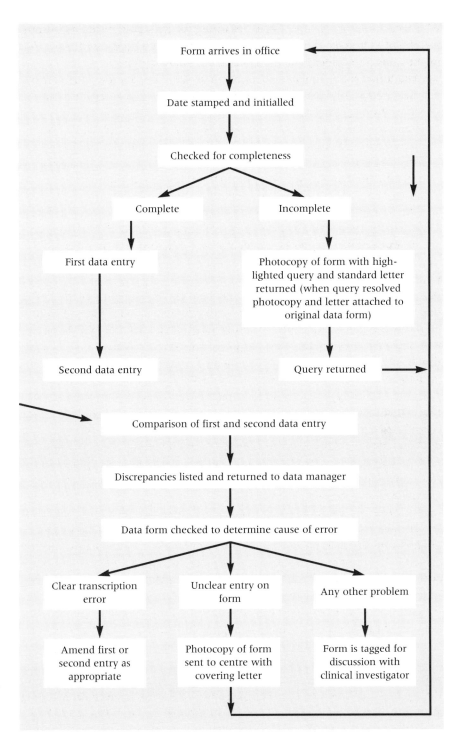

Figure 14.1 Handling data for research projects

written answers word for word and specialised software packages are available to assist in this type of work. Do consider using one of these packages if it is warranted, as it can assist you in the analysis of your project. Quantitative research however, is unlikely to require lengthy text answers and most data can be coded for ease of analysis. By coding, we mean that a text response is given a code which makes it easier to handle at the analysis stage. For example, if you are asking about use of analgesia then you might want to use '1' for aspirin, '2' for paracetamol, '3' for codeine, and so on. Using the numeric code instead of the text means that misspelling, etc. becomes less important. Additionally, it is simpler to load numeric data into a computer database.

Distinguishing missing data from data that are unknown

It is at this time that a distinction should be made between data indicated as 'unknown' by the person completing the form – that is, the piece of information you are requesting was never collected and hence is not known – and data which are 'missing' – that is, information you have requested does exist, but the person completing the form either cannot or will not find it. This allows you to make a judgement about the benefit of including a question that may have (for example) a 65% response rate of 'unknown' but a 'missing' response rate of only 5%. Similarly, if a question requires the person answering it to find information elsewhere, you may have a very high 'missing' rate and the question therefore may be deemed unsuitable. This is the benefit of pilot studies, which allow you to determine all this before commencing a large project.

Data collection – electronic or paper format?

How do you decide if your data should be collected and analysed on paper or electronically? There are clear benefits and disadvantages in each case. In the case of electronic data collection, the data are entered immediately, at source, into a computer and the data saved on disk. This is quick and has the benefit of requiring very little physical storage space. However, it can be very difficult to decide how to handle unexpected responses when you are sitting in front of the computer and the respondent is waiting for you to move on to the next question. In addition, information entered directly into a computer cannot be verified and usually cannot be double-entered unless this is done twice at the point of origin (see later for more details about double entry).

In the case of data collection on paper, there is a clear disadvantage in terms of physical storage space required. However, there are many benefits of paper data collection. The first is that you have a permanent paper record of the answer to a question, to which any queries may be referred. In addition, data entry can be conducted at convenient times and if the answer to a question appears incorrect, this can be checked by returning a copy to the person responsible for completing it. On balance, paper data collection (with subsequent entry on to computer if appropriate) tends to be more accurate. The combination of the two, with paper and electronic backup disks gives most flexibility and minimises data loss.

Staff

So who is doing all this work? The number of staff you employ to conduct a project will depend entirely on the amount of data being collected. If the project is relatively small and has very little money, it may be that you will do everything yourself. In this case, every effort should be made to find some-body else willing to do second data entry for you so that the accuracy of your data set will not be challenged. At the other extreme are very large randomised controlled trials. Some of these trials may require you to collect data from thousands of subjects and will need staff to run the project efficiently.

There are several options you can consider in terms of staff for a large project. In the case of electronic data being collected at source, at least two people will need to be identified in each centre collecting data, in order to do double data entry, and a computer programmer may be needed to set up the initial systems and prepare data for analysis. No further staff are necessary – any missing data in this system remain missing forever, as there are no paper copies to return to respondents with requests for further information. In the case of paper data collection you could consider employing a data manager, whose job it is to ensure that the data set is as complete and accurate as possible and who is in charge of following up all missing data. If you wish, the data manager could also be responsible for first data entry – this will depend on the size of the project. A second person to conduct second data entry will also be needed, as well as a computer programmer. If the project is very large, two data entry clerks may be needed in addition to the data manager in order to complete the data entry.

Preparing for analysis

Finally, you should consider how to handle the analysis of your data. Should this be on paper (only for a small project) or have you entered the data into a custom-designed computer database, spreadsheet or other software package? For a large project, you might also consider specialised scanning software which would enable you to scan your data forms. As prices fall and software/hardware becomes more accurate this has become a more realistic option.

If you have entered the data into a computer then, as stated previously, we would strongly recommend using double data entry to minimise typograph-ical errors, difficulties of interpretation of illegible handwriting, and so on. The two sets of data should have been entered by two different people on two separate occasions without conferring. In terms of discrepancies between first and second data entry, there are two options. If you have a customised data entry program then, at the time of second entry, an error message could appear on the screen if a discrepancy is noted by the computer program. This message informs the second data entry person that the value just entered is different from the value entered by the first person. The second data entry person can then check the paper copy and make a decision as to the correct answer. The disadvantage of this system is that the person doing second data entry is unlikely to be qualified to make such decisions. For example, if it is a clinical question, then it should be referred to the appropriate person. Therefore, a second option is that a printout of discrepancies can be produced after all data entry. Computer software is available which will do this. This list is presented to the appropriate person, who can make decisions based on whether the discrepancy is due to a simple error at the time of data entry, an error due to unclear handwriting (which may need to be verified with the person completing the form) or an error due to any other reason.

Any annotations to data forms should be in a different coloured ink, should not obliterate the original entry and must be initialled and dated by the data manager or principal investigator. An additional safeguard is to have an 'audit trail' built into your computer program so that any changes to the data are recorded with the initials of the person making the change and the date, and so that changes can be followed through later. This has overheads in terms of computer disk space required but is well worth doing if at all possible.

Storing and backing-up data

Finally, perhaps the most crucial element of your research is the backing-up of your data. There are often plaintive advertisements in the newspapers: 'Lost/stolen, laptop computer containing the only record of x years' work'. Do not put yourself in this position. After spending considerable time and energy obtaining a complete data set, you do not want to lose it due to a computer malfunction or theft. *All* data should be backed-up on a very regular basis – certainly not less often than weekly and preferably daily – and the backup stored in a separate location. You can back-up your data manually on to floppy disks or purchase backup software in the case of a larger study. You should remove at least one copy of the data from the building in which the original data set is held and update this copy regularly. In addition, you must make sure that you can restore your data from the backup disks. All too often, the crucial backups are found to be unusable at the very time they are needed.

In conclusion, the systems used to ensure good data management are not complex – but they are important. Thinking about these systems at the outset of your project will save you a great deal of time and energy and should ensure that you gather the best possible data, resulting in a far better research project. Good luck!

15

Statistics

Peter Brocklehurst
and Simon Gates

In this chapter we aim to give a basic introduction to the main concepts involved in planning and undertaking statistical analysis and to indicate what methods of analysis should be used in common situations. We do not give details of how to carry out the statistical tests; these can be found in many statistics textbooks and a list of suitable reference books is provided at the end of the chapter. The examples used to illustrate some of the statistical concepts are predominantly clinical studies, but the concepts apply equally to other research settings, such as laboratory-based studies.

Why we need statistics

Statistics are necessary because of the intrinsic variability of humans and animals. Every individual who could be included in a research study is different and will respond differently to an intervention or exposure to a risk factor. A group of subjects who experience the same intervention or risk factor will, therefore, not all respond in the same way, but there will be a range of responses. In a research study, we usually want to discover if there is a difference between two or more groups of individuals who have been given different treatments or have experienced different exposures. The individuals in each group will differ just by chance, so in each group there will be a range of responses. To find out whether the different treatments have any effect on the outcome we need to separate the effects of chance variation from those of the treatment. Statistical methods provide ways of doing this: they help us to understand the relationships between variables and to draw valid conclusions.

What statistical methods are used for

Statistical methods are used for three purposes:

- Summarising data for presentation, by means of summary statistics and graphs. Summary statistics measure the central characteristic of a set of data and the spread around it, for example by the mean and standard deviation or the median and interquartile range.
- Finding out how likely it is that the data obtained in a study could have arisen by chance and, hence, how likely it is that there is a real difference between the groups studied.
- Assessing the reliability of results and generalising from the individuals in

the study to the whole population of which they are part. For example, if a study is carried out on 100 pregnant women, the result will depend partly on the characteristics of these women and would be slightly different if a different set of 100 women were selected. Statistical methods enable us to assess how well the result from the individuals in the study represents the whole of the population from which they are drawn.

Quantitative and qualitative research

In broad terms, quantitative research is concerned with enumeration; for example, measuring whether an exposure leads to an outcome and, if so, by how much that outcome is increased, or measuring the size of an effect of a new intervention. Qualitative research is concerned more with why social factors lead to changes in outcome or how an intervention is effective. For example, if a smoking cessation programme in pregnancy is to be evaluated, quantitative methods can be used to assess how effective the programme is (by carrying out an RCT). Qualitative methods, such as interview studies, can be used to explore why the intervention works and what aspects of it change women's perceptions of the risks they and their babies face by continuing to smoke.

Planning statistical analyses

The key to easy and successful analysis is planning. Before data collection is started, it is essential to know:

- what data will be collected and what will then be done with them
- what comparisons will be made and what statistical procedures will be used.

Without adequate planning, you run the risk of failing to collect all of the necessary data, or of wasting effort on gathering data that are impossible to analyse. Collecting data is difficult and expensive, so it pays to be clear at the outset exactly what data will be collected and what will not.

Writing a study protocol is essential. This should contain as much detail as possible on:

- what data will be collected
- the methods of data collection
- sample size calculations (see Chapter 10)
- methods of analysis.

The analysis is an important part of the project, so it should be included in the plan which is drawn up at the start. You should discuss the study while you are planning it with researchers and statisticians who have experience in the type of study design and analytical methods that you propose to use. At this stage, you can make changes to your plans in the light of other people's experience and expertise.

Types of data

The type of analysis that is done will depend on what questions are to be asked and on the types of data that have been collected. Different sorts of data require different sorts of analysis and you should be careful not to use statistical tests that are inappropriate for your data, as doing so may give erroneous results.

Continuous variables are those which are measured on a continuous scale, such as height and weight. Discrete variables can take only certain values, such as the number of cases of a disease in a week, which can only be a whole number. Categorical variables are ones where each individual is in one of a number of mutually exclusive classes, such as country of birth, sex or type of drug. Categorical variables may be ordered, where the categories form a natural sequence. For example, the number of children a woman has is an ordered categorical, whereas country of birth is not ordered. Binary variables are an important type of categorical variable, where there are only two classes such as yes or no, alive or dead, preterm or term.

For many variables, if a plot is made of each value against its frequency in a large number of people, the resulting graph will have a characteristic symmetrical bell shape. Birth weight is an example of such a variable; the most common value is the mean birth weight and the majority of people have a birth weight fairly close to this. Extremely high or low birth weights are much rarer. A plot such as this of the frequency of occurrence of each possible value shows the distribution of the data and the symmetrical bell-shaped curve is known as a normal distribution. There are many possible distributions of data; some examples are shown in Figure 15.1. The distribution of the data is important because it affects the way the analysis is done. Some statistical methods require that the data are sampled from a normal distribution (see parametric statistics, below) and, if this is not the case, other methods should be used.

It can sometimes be more meaningful to present continuous data as categorical variables. For example, suppose that, in an RCT comparing two operative techniques, the mean blood loss was 435 ml in the group given the new treatment, and 389 ml in the conventional treatment group. If the question of interest is whether the patients had any major blood loss, these figures are uninformative. An alternative way of presenting the same data would be to calculate the proportion of patients in each group who lost more than 500 ml at operation: 41% in the new treatment group and 38% in the conventional treatment group. How to present data depends on what information the investigators wish to convey and a continuous outcome sometimes fails to convey the relevant information.

The outcome which is being measured is often referred to as the response variable, to distinguish it from the explanatory variable or variables. For example, in an experiment comparing two drug treatments for hypertension in pregnancy, the response variable would be blood pressure and the explana-

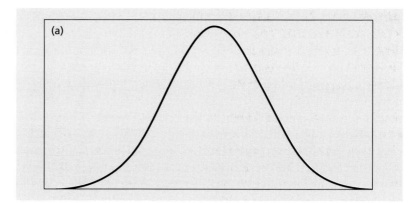

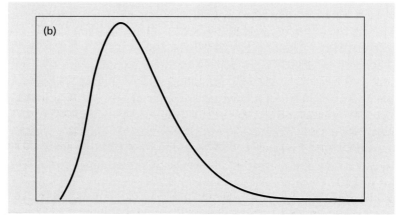

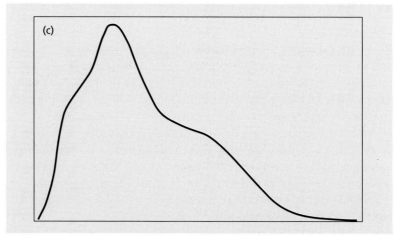

Figure 15.1 Some examples of distributions of variables: (a) a normal distribution; (b) a non-normal distribution; this one is asymmetrical, with a 'tail' on the right; (c) a different non-normal distribution; this one has a complex shape

tory variable would be a categorical variable with two classes, one for each drug.

Risks and odds

Binary response variables, where each individual has one of two possible outcomes, are usually presented as risks or odds. These are ways of summarising the data and making comparisons between groups. The risk is the proportion of the group under study who develop the outcome of interest. For instance, if 1000 primigravid women are followed throughout their pregnancy and 20 of them develop gestational diabetes, the risk of developing gestational diabetes in this group is 20/1000 or 2%.

The odds is the ratio of the number of a group who develop the outcome of interest to the number who do not. Using the example above, the odds of developing gestational diabetes are 20/(1000–20) = 20/980 = 2.04%.

As this example demonstrates, when the outcome is uncommon, the odds are very similar to the risk. Odds rather than risks have to be used where the total population at risk is not known, so a risk cannot be calculated; for example, in case–control studies (see Chapter 16).

The most common use for odds or risks is in comparisons of two groups; a ratio of the odds (the odds ratio – OR) or risk (relative risk – RR) between the two groups is calculated and this gives a measure of the difference between the groups. Confidence intervals can be calculated for the OR or RR and results are commonly presented in this way (see Comparing proportions, below).

As an example of the calculation of the OR and RR, consider an RCT investigating the effects of two different antibiotic regimens for the prevention of postoperative infection. A table can be constructed (Table 15.1). From this the odds ratio and the relative risk can be calculated:

Odds ratio = Odds of infection with antibiotic A
       Odds of infection with antibiotic B

      = (Infections with antibiotic A/No infections with antibiotic A)
        (Infections with antibiotic B/No infections with antibiotic B)

      = 23/85
        40/66

      = 0.45

Relative risk = Risk of infection with A
       Risk of infection with B

      = (Number infected with antibiotic A/Total number given antibiotic A)
        (Number infected with antibiotic B/Total number given antibiotic B)

      = 23/(85+23)
        40/(66+40)

      = 0.56

Table 15.1 A table to calculate the OR and RR		
	Infections	**No infections**
Antibiotic A	23	85
Antibiotic B	40	66

The interpretation of these results is that antibiotic A is associated with a halving of the incidence of postoperative infection compared with antibiotic B.

Concepts involved in statistical analysis

Confidence intervals
Because the individuals included in a research study are a sample from a larger population, it is important to know how well the study's results reflect the true value for the whole population. For example, a study might be carried out on 100 pregnant women. How well does the result for these women match the result that would be obtained if all pregnant women could be studied? Confidence intervals provide a way of measuring the reliability of results, by giving a range around the result within which you would reasonably expect the true value for the population to lie. If the confidence interval is wide, there is a wide range of values which the true value could be, so the result is a poor estimate of it. If the confidence interval is narrow, the result measures the true value in the population fairly precisely. Usually 95% confidence intervals are calculated, which give a range that will include the true value with a probability of 0.95.

Hypothesis testing
Hypothesis testing is the process by which we can ask how likely it is that an observed result is due to chance alone. To do this, a wide variety of statistical tests exist, which all work in the same basic way: they work out how likely it is that the observed data would have been obtained if there were really no difference between the groups. The hypothesis that there is no difference is known as the null hypothesis. Statistical tests express this likelihood as a probability, known as the *P* value. A high *P* value means that you can accept the null hypothesis and conclude that there is no difference between your groups. If the *P* value is low, you can reject the null hypothesis and conclude that there is a real difference. The convention has arisen of using a *P* value of 0.05 as the cut-off for whether two groups are considered 'significantly' different. This means that the existence of a real difference is concluded if the probability is less than 0.05, or in other words, if there is less than a 1 in 20 chance that the result is due simply to random variation.

The main problem with *P* values is that they tell you nothing about the size of the difference between the groups. If the sample size is very large, a *P* value of less than 0.05 can result from a very small and clinically unimportant difference. Conversely, if the sample size is small, a large and potentially clinically important difference may yield a *P* value of greater than 0.05. For this reason, it is not recommended to present results simply as *P* values. It is much more informative to present an estimate of the size of the difference between groups together with a confidence interval.

Power

Statistical tests are not completely reliable and there is a chance that a test will fail to discover a real difference, even though there is one. The probability that a test will discover a real difference is called its power. Power is influenced by sample size and by the size of the difference – a larger difference will be easier to detect and will give the test more power, as will a larger sample size. Failure to find a difference between two groups may be because none exists, or it may be because of lack of power in the test. It is important to consider statistical power in planning what sample size is necessary in your study; the study must be large enough to give the test used sufficient power to provide an answer to the question being investigated.

Parametric and non-parametric statistics

Statistical tests can be broadly divided into parametric and non-parametric tests. The essential difference between them is that parametric statistics make assumptions about the distribution of the data, as they involve calculating parameters from the data, whereas non-parametric statistics do not (hence their alternative name 'distribution-free statistics'). If you use parametric statistics, it is important that their assumptions are met; if not, or if there is doubt about this, non-parametric statistics should be preferred. One of the most common assumptions of parametric statistics is that the data should be normally distributed. Many common measurements, such as length of post-surgical hospital stay, operating time and duration of labour, are not normally distributed; their distributions are asymmetrical because there are a few people for which these durations are very long. In these cases, either non-parametric methods should be used or the data should be transformed. Transformation simply means subjecting all of the values of the response variable to some mathematical operation, such as taking logarithms, so that the data become normally distributed. If the transformation is successful, they can then be analysed using parametric methods. Alternatively, continuous data can be changed to a categorical variable (for example, the length of stay in hospital after hysterectomy could be changed to the number of women in hospital for more than seven days after their operation) and the groups can then be compared using parametric methods.

Carrying out statistical analyses

Exploratory analysis

The first step in an analysis should be to familiarise yourself with the data, by calculating summary statistics, creating tables and plotting graphs. If you are comparing a normally distributed continuous variable between two groups, the mean and standard deviation (SD) for each group should be calculated. With a non-normally distributed continuous variable, the median value represents the central characteristic of the data and the interquartile range represents its spread. If you are looking for an association between two continuous variables, plot the two variables against each other. If your response variable is categorical, tables of counts and proportions are appropriate.

These exploratory steps will help you to see any features of the data which were not anticipated that you may need to explore further in your analysis. For example, you may have anticipated a linear relationship between two continuous variables. However, a graph of the data may suggest that it is actually curved. This can then be incorporated into the analysis; you can carry out a test to see if a curve fits the data better than a straight line. Furthermore, this sort of examination of the data can highlight any errors in the data and reveal any data points that look very different from the rest (known as 'outliers'). These should be investigated carefully: has something atypical happened to those individuals, or have the data not been recorded correctly?

Statistical software

Virtually all analyses are done by computer and many large and comprehensive software packages (such as SAS, SPSS, Stata and Minitab) are available. These can give you all of the statistics you are likely to need. Which to use is largely a matter of personal preference.

There are two common problems with statistical software:

- They will often produce answers uncritically, even if the analysis you are running is inappropriate. The computer can do complicated calculations easily, but the analyst still needs to know what he or she is doing.
- Their output can be very confusing, sometimes producing pages of output from a simple test. Manuals supplied with the software may be unhelpful, so it is advisable to refer to someone who is experienced with the software you propose to use.

Methods of analysis

Comparing means

When a study compares two groups in which the outcome is a continuous variable, the means of the two groups can be compared. For example, in a study comparing birth weight in two groups of babies, the mean of the first group of 206 babies is 3254 g (SD 438 g) and that of the other group of 184 babies is 3602 g (SD 509 g). There are several ways of comparing these data and the method used will depend on what information the investigators wish to convey. If the purpose is to demonstrate that the difference between the two groups is unlikely to have occurred by chance, then a t test will produce a *P* value (for this example, the *P* value is less than 0.001, so this difference in birth weight is unlikely to have occurred by chance). However, to determine not only whether a difference exists but to find out how large it is, then the difference in mean birth weight can be calculated, together with a confidence interval, which expresses the uncertainty around the estimate of the difference. In this example, the difference between the means is 348 g, 95% confidence interval 254–442 g. Therefore, the difference between the birth weights of these two groups of women is between 254 g and 442 g. This is unlikely to have occurred by chance, as the range does not include 0 or a negative value.

Another way to compare these data would be to compare the incidence of low birth weight (less than 2500 g) in each group; that is, to convert birth weight into a categorical variable.

The non-parametric equivalent of the t test is the Mann–Whitney test.

Comparing more than two means
If there are more than two groups to be compared, the approach used will depend on what information the investigators wish to convey. If there are four groups of women and each group has a mean postoperative haemoglobin, then comparing each of three groups with one 'baseline' group (which would usually be the control treatment) may be the approach which is adopted. This will yield three *P* values or three mean differences, each with a 95% confidence interval (as above). Alternatively, the investigators may simply want to investigate whether the four groups are different from each other, in which case an analysis of variance (ANOVA) can be performed and a *P* value will result. If a non-parametric test is needed, the Mann–Whitney tests can be used for pair-wise comparisons, and the Kruskal–Wallis test is the equivalent of the ANOVA.

Comparing proportions
If the outcome is measured as a binary variable, the proportion of individuals who have it in each group can be compared. As with comparing means, different methods can be used depending on the question being addressed. If the aim is to determine whether the two proportions are different and whether this difference is unlikely to be due to chance then a χ^2 (chi-square) test is appropriate and will yield a *P* value. However, if the aim is to estimate how different two proportions are then the difference between them and a 95% confidence interval for this difference can be presented. Alternatively, the odds ratio or risk ratio between the two groups with its 95% confidence interval can be calculated.

For example, an RCT which aims to determine the proportion of women who continue to experience climacteric symptoms with a new treatment finds that 20% (124/620) of women in the standard treatment group have persistent symptoms compared with 11% (66/598) in the new treatment group. Is this different?

A χ^2 test produces a *P* value of < 0.001, suggesting that the difference is unlikely to be due to chance. The difference in proportions is 9%, with a 95% confidence interval of 5–13%, suggesting that 5–13% fewer women in the new treatment group have persistent symptoms. The odds ratio is 0.50, with a 95% confidence interval of 0.35–0.69, suggesting that women in the new treatment group are between 35% and 69% less likely to have persistent symptoms than those in the standard treatment group.

When comparing proportions between the groups of an ordered categorical variable, for example birth weight groups, a test-for-trend can be performed (in some software packages, this is found under analysis of variance). This will produce a *P* value and will demonstrate whether the distribution of birth weights within the two groups of women is different. The advantage of comparing groups using a test-for-trend is an increase in the power of the test to detect more modest differences than a simple comparison of two groups (for example, < 2500 g and ≥ 2500 g).

Association between continuous variables

If both the explanatory and response variables are continuous, they can be analysed by correlation (Figure 15.2) or linear regression (Figure 15.3). Which of these to use depends on the question being asked. Regression supposes that the response variable depends on the explanatory variable and produces an equation relating them and a *P* value. Correlation does not assume that one variable causes the other, but simply measures their association, by means of a correlation coefficient. This can be between −1 and +1, with 0 representing no association, −1 perfect negative association and +1 perfect positive association. Perfect correlation does not always mean perfect agreement. Consider a comparison of two methods for measuring neonatal bilirubin. There may be perfect correlation but one test may always produce a lower reading than the other. There are both parametric and non-parametric correlation coefficients. The non-parametric version uses a ranking of the data rather than the actual values.

Confounding

Accounting for confounding (see Chapter 16) in the analysis of a study can be performed using stratification or multiple regression analysis.

Stratification, at its simplest, involves setting up two-by-two tables for each level of the confounding variable. For example, when trying to determine whether coffee drinking in pregnancy is associated with preterm delivery the following results table may be constructed (Table 15.2).

A potential confounder of this association could be cigarette smoking and

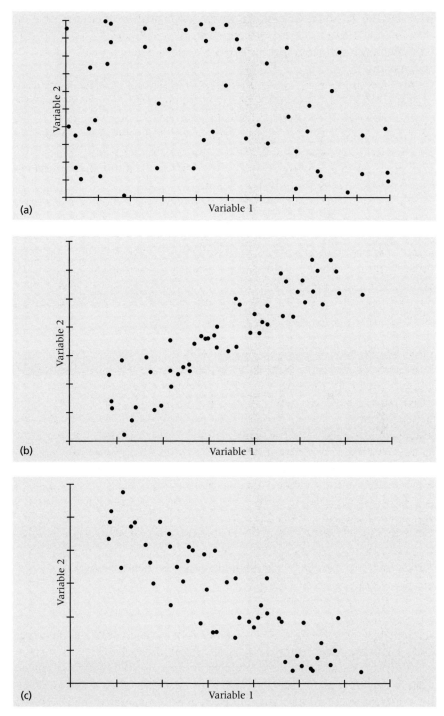

Figure 15.2 Examples of correlations between two variables: (a) correlation coefficient of zero; (b) a positive correlation; (c) a negative correlation

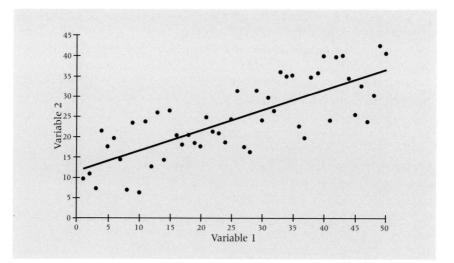

Figure 15.3 A linear regression. The regression procedure calculates a best-fit line through the data, and produces the equation of this line and a *P* value

Table 15.2 The association between coffee drinking and preterm delivery		
	Preterm delivery	**Term delivery**
Coffee drinkers	36	364
Non-coffee drinkers	39	560
Odds ratio = 1.9		

Table 15.3 Smokers versus non-smokers		
Smokers:	**Preterm delivery**	**Term delivery**
Coffee drinkers	17	120
Non-coffee drinkers	12	97
Odds ratio = 1.2		
Non-smokers:	**Preterm delivery**	**Term delivery**
Coffee drinkers	19	244
Non-coffee drinkers	27	463
Odds ratio = 1.3		

the analysis can be stratified by whether the women smoked during their pregnancy or not. In reality, smoking status is usually split into more detailed levels but, for the purposes of illustration, the variable will be divided into 'yes' and 'no'. Another table (Table 15.3) can now be constructed.

The results from the stratified tables can be combined using, for example, the Mantel–Haenszel method. This will produce a summary OR of the association between coffee drinking and preterm delivery which has been 'adjusted' for smoking. Stratified analyses are straightforward to carry out and simple to understand, but cannot control for more than a small number of confounders at one time. Where it is necessary to control for several confounders simultaneously multi-variate analyses can be used, of which the most common is multiple regression analysis. The main problem with this technique is that, as the calculations have to be carried out by computer, the data can be simply fed into the 'model' and a result appears without any clear understanding of the data or the modelling process. The properties of the data and the way the model is constructed can affect the results and, for this reason, multiple regression analysis should only be attempted under close supervision by a statistician experienced with this method.

Meta-analysis

The results of individual studies are subject to the same sort of random variation as affects individual subjects within studies. When several studies have addressed the same question, it is desirable that their results should be summarised in some way and the overall result from all of the studies estimated. This should give a more accurate estimate of the true effect than can be gained from any individual study. The statistical methods for combining studies in this way are known as 'meta-analysis'. Several methods exist for carrying out such analyses. In essence, the methods are similar to stratification mentioned above, but the strata (the individual studies) are weighted by some measures, usually the size of the study. It is crucial to the success of meta-analysis that all existing studies are included. Basing the analysis only on well-known studies is likely to introduce bias, as studies showing a large effect may be more likely to be published or widely publicised.

Bayesian analysis

Bayesian analysis is a different approach to statistical analysis. It aims to incorporate into the analysis what was known or believed before the study began and it produces a composite result, combining what has been observed in the study with previous knowledge. Previous knowledge is represented as a probability distribution (the 'prior distribution'), which shows the probability of the possible outcomes. This is modified by the new data to produce a new distribution (the 'posterior distribution'), which represents the probability of the range of outcomes given the information from both sets of data. Bayesian analysis is becoming more widely used, but is still controversial.

Further reading

Abelson, R.P. (1995) *Statistics as Principled Argument*. Hillsdale, NJ: Lawrence Erlbaum Associates

Altman, D.G. (1991) *Practical Statistics for Medical Research*. London: Chapman and Hall

Bland, M. (1995) *An Introduction to Medical Statistics*. Oxford: Oxford University Press

Gardner, M.J. and Altman, D.G. (1989) *Statistics With Confidence*. London: BMJ Publishing Group

Kirkwood, B.R. (1988) *Essentials of Medical Statistics*. Oxford: Blackwell Scientific Publications

Swinscow, T.D.V. (1980) *Statistics at Square One*, 7th edn. London: British Medical Association

## 16

Epidemiology

Paul B. Silcocks

What is epidemiology?

Loosely speaking, epidemiology is the study of diseases in defined populations. In some ways it can be thought of as the population equivalent of pathology in the individual, but epidemiology is also a branch of applied statistics – motivated by practical medical problems. While numeracy is important, it is not necessary to have a degree in mathematics to contribute to the subject or to derive benefit from an epidemiological approach to medicine.

Branches of epidemiology

Descriptive

Descriptive epidemiology provides general statements on the occurrence of disease by attributes such as age, sex, occupation, class, race, geographic location and calendar period. This information is basic to public health and hypothesis generation. Sources of information include routinely available mortality statistics and cancer registrations and also the results of *ad hoc* surveys.

Analytic

'Analytic' epidemiological studies test ideas relating to the cause, classification, diagnosis or outcome of a disease. Examples are whether smoking causes cervical cancer, how the performance of cytological screening can be evaluated and what factors influence survival. The randomised controlled trial (RCT) can be thought of as a very specialised instance of analytic epidemiology.

Theoretical

Theoretical epidemiology is based on mathematical models to simulate disease occurrence – normally implemented on a computer. Such simulations may indicate which public health interventions are likely to be most effective, or show where additional evidence needs to be acquired. Examples are models of the AIDS epidemic, screening programmes for cancer and carcinogenesis. A very early example – from 1760 – is Daniel Bernouilli's study on the effects of smallpox vaccination. We will not consider this branch any further.

Clinical epidemiology

Clinical epidemiology is that part of the discipline applied to patients and clinical problems, rather than the population as a whole.

Concepts

The key concepts in epidemiology relate to risk. Risk is the probability of an *event* occurring. 'Risk' and 'probability' are used interchangeably. In a sample of individuals we can estimate risk of death as the proportion of individuals who die. We say that the number originally alive is the number *at risk*.

$$\text{Risk} = \frac{\text{Deaths}}{\text{Population at risk}}$$

However, if 12 out of a class of 30 school children die in two years, it is more worrying than if this occurred over sixty years.

'Rates' can be thought of as risk per unit of time, so the denominator is person-time, which distinguishes a rate from a risk (typically this is expressed as *x* cases per 100 000 per year).

$$\text{Risk} = \frac{\text{Deaths}}{\text{Person-time at risk}}$$

'Person-time' is simply the sum of the times for which each individual in the population at risk is observed: one person living for one year equals one person-year; two persons living for six months equals one person-year; one person living for one year plus one living for two years equals three person-years.

For short periods and/or small risk, the rate approximates the risk. If the event is death (as above) this is termed a 'mortality rate'. If the event is a new diagnosis of disease, it is an 'incidence rate'. Incidence is simply the number of newly diagnosed cases in a given periond. An 'age-specific rate' refers to a specific age group (e.g. 35–39 year olds). Sex and social class-specific rates can be defined analogously.

'Odds' are another way of looking at risk. There is no mystery about odds and there is a 1:1 relationship between risk and odds:

$$\text{Odds} = \frac{\text{Risk}}{(1 - \text{Risk})}$$

We can easily convert odds to risk using:

$$\text{Risk} = \frac{\text{Odds}}{(1 + \text{Odds})}$$

Odds are sometimes more easily handled than risks.

We can compare risks of disease in two groups using the ratio of the risks, the ratio of the rates or the ratio of the odds. Since these mathematically distinct measures are numerically very close for small risks, they are often referred to loosely as 'relative risk' – which, strictly, means just the risk ratio.

'Prevalence' is the number of cases alive with the disease either at a single point in time (point prevalence) or over a defined period (period prevalence). When these values are divided by the population size, we obtain point and period prevalence 'rates' (actually not rates but proportions).

If the duration of the disease and its incidence rate are not changing over time, then:

Incidence rate × Duration = Prevalence 'rate' (approximately).

Descriptive epidemiology

The basic sources for descriptive epidemiology of disease are either *ad hoc* surveys or routinely available information in the form of official statistics published by the Office of National Statistics (ONS), formerly the Office of Population Censuses and Surveys (OPCS).

Population size is needed to obtain prevalence, incidence and mortality rates. This is obtained from the decennial census. Between censuses, the ONS provides the population estimates by subtracting deaths, adding births and allowing for emigrants, although these may be miscounted and the homeless may be missed.

Mortality

The registration of death has been compulsory since 1874 and mortality data tend to be of reasonably good quality (misclassification of death notwith-standing). Death certificates have an internationally agreed structure with Part I listing the immediate cause of death and conditions leading to it from which the underlying cause is coded. Other significant conditions contributing to the death are noted in Part II. The underlying cause is what appears in routine mortality statistics, but the other causes are coded at the ONS.

For rapidly fatal diseases, the place and time of death is almost as good as place and time of diagnosis. Mortality data also offer complete population coverage, a clear end point and long usage. Disadvantages are inaccuracy (in the elderly), an incomplete account of multiple pathology and inapplicability to non-fatal disease occurrence. Other important end-points such as quality of life and resource use are also missed.

Summarising mortality

When comparing disease mortality or incidence rates between different parts of the country, or between occupation groups, allowance needs to be made for variation in the age structure of the groups under study. Such unadjusted rates are termed 'crude rates'. The effect of age can be allowed for by age-standardisation, to yield 'age-adjusted' or 'age-standardised rates'.

There are two basic methods: direct and indirect standardisation, but the details are not important here. The key point is that, as age varies with the groups under study and as the disease rate varies with age, this is basically a problem of confounding and standardisation is just another form of stratified analysis. Standardisation for sex and class is also possible.

Alternatives for mortality statistics are to present the cumulative risk of death from a disease ('lifetime' risk – actually to age 74) or to present a 'current life' table. This depicts what the survival of a single birth cohort would be if it experienced present day mortality rates at each age.

Such life tables are used to estimate expectation of life from any age and are the basis for insurance, pension schemes and population forecasts. Variation between regions in expectation of life from birth has been shown to be greater than the effect of cancer (Gardner and Donnan 1977).

Male and female life tables for Trent are displayed in Figure 16.1 and show, for example, that median survival from birth is about five years greater in women than men. English life tables are available in series DH1 (Table 16.1).

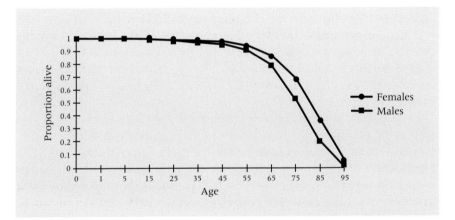

Figure 16.1 Trent life table (1991)

Table 16.1 Routinely available statistics on disease produced by the Office for National Statistics	
Topic	**Series**
Population size	VS
Mortality	
General	DH1
Cause	DH2
Area	DH5
Cancer	MB1
Communicable disease	MB2
Congenital malformations	MB3
General practice	MB5

Morbidity

The most specific, accurate and complete routinely collected morbidity data are on cancer. The England and Wales National Cancer Registry, run by ONS, probably holds the largest registry data set on cancers in the world. It has been estimated that the total data set now contains about five million cancers from a population of about 1500 million person-years at risk.

Cancer registration is not a statutory obligation. Data collection is organised through regional registries, which submit a standard data set to ONS. The origins of the system lie in hospital-based registries which began in the 1920s. Since 1947, the General Register Office (now part of ONS) has taken on this responsibility.

The main disease-related routine statistics are listed in Table 16.1. Routinely available health-related information includes hospital episode statistics, the General Household Survey (questions on sickness-limited activity, visits to doctors and hospitals and smoking and drinking habits), the National Food Survey (information on food purchases at regional level), the Family Spending Survey (expenditure on food and tobacco).

A complete list of sources of routinely collected information is given in the *Guide to Official Statistics* (HMSO 1996).

Routine statistics delineate the north-south, urban-rural and social class variations in mortality, as well as being the basis for numerous descriptive and analytic epidemiological studies.

Analytic epidemiology

Aetiology

We actually observe only the conjunction of events, from which we must infer cause. We can extend the concept of cause to events that are only 'probable', by looking for association. Association is when events occur together more, or less, often than one would expect.

In epidemiology, association is typically measured by the difference in risk of disease between:

- exposed and unexposed (excess risk)
- the ratio of the risk in exposed to the risk in unexposed (relative risk)
- the ratio of the odds of disease in exposed to the odds in unexposed (odds ratio).

If no association is present the excess risk will be 0 and the relative risk (and odds ratio) will be 1.

The difficulty is whether an association is causal (recognising that most diseases are multifactorial and that causes may operate by predisposing an individual to a disease, precipitating its onset or aggravating its course). Pragmatic criteria for accepting an association as causal in observational studies were suggested by Bradford Hill (1952):

- consistency of association – results are replicated in studies using different methods, in a variety of settings
- strength of association – the larger the magnitude of the excess risk or relative risk the more persuasive the evidence
- specificity – when a suspected cause produces a single well defined effect
- dose/response relationship – when increasing the exposure produces larger excess or relative risks
- time sequence – the exposure must have preceded the event
- biological plausibility – when the association makes biological sense
- coherence – for example, if the association 'explains' other facts known about the disease, such as age and sex distribution
- experiment – if removal of the cause reduces the risk of disease.

Ways of establishing association

We can do this by means of intervention studies (i.e. experiment, including RCTs) or by observational studies – using either the cohort or the case–control approach. For any of these, the units or subjects of study may be at an ecological or individual level.

An example of an ecological level observational study is the correlation of breast cancer mortality rates and average fat consumption in different countries. For intervention studies, an example would be the reduction in cervical cancer mortality rates following the introduction of a screening programme. Ecological level studies also arise in the context of RCTs as 'cluster randomised' studies.

The weakness of ecological level studies is that associations found at group level need not appear when individuals are studied. This is called the ecologic fallacy. Ecological level studies are useful to generate hypotheses and are appropriate if the proposed intervention will be applied anyway in a mass fashion (such as legislation).

The RCT is probably the kind of intervention study most familiar to clinicians and it can be summarised as follows:

- Aim:
  — does ovarian cancer respond better to Taxol than to conventional chemotherapy?
- Method:
  — choose suitable patients
  — randomise to Taxol and control groups
  — measure percentage responding
- Result:
  — Taxol group has greater percentage of responders (or not).
  — The key point is that subjects are alike, apart from the exposure of interest.

The cohort study is basically the same, except that crucially allocation to the exposure is no longer under the investigator's control:

- Aim:
  - does smoking cause cervical cancer?
- Method:
  - choose subjects without cervical cancer
  - identify smokers and non-smokers
  - follow them over time
- Result:
  - greater percentage of cervical cancer cases in smokers (maybe).

Both the RCT and the cohort study can be depicted in a 2 × 2 table (Table 16.2). In practice, the results are likely to be expressed as rates rather than risks, with person-time as the denominator, but as rates can be converted to risks and hence odds, this does not affect the argument.

Case–control studies appear at first sight to be different, since the answer to the smoking question is obtained in a 'back to front' manner and the probabilities of previous exposure are compared, not the risks of getting the disease:

- Aim:
  - does smoking cause lung cancer?
- Method:
  - choose subjects
  - identify cervical cancer cases and controls (without cervical cancer)
  - ask about past smoking
- Result:
  - greater percentage of smokers in cervical cancer patients.

However, looking at the corresponding 2 × 2 table (Table 16.3), it can be seen that the relative odds of exposure are the same as the relative odds of disease which would have been obtained from a cohort study (provided the disease was rare). Thus, while the case–control study cannot estimate relative risk directly (you sample cases and controls), provided the disease is rare, the odds ratio you get from a case–control study approximates the relative risk which you would have obtained from a cohort.

Table 16.2 RCTs and cohort studies

	Become ill	Do not become ill	Total
Exposed	a	b	a + b
Unexposed	c	d	c + d

$$\text{Relative risk of disease} = \frac{a/(a + b)}{c/(c + d)}$$

$$\equiv \frac{ad}{bc} \quad \text{if the disease is rare (when } a \ll b \text{ and } c \ll d\text{)}$$

Table 16.3 Case–control studies			
	Become ill	**Do not become ill**	**Total**
Exposed	a	b	a + b
Unexposed	c	d	c + d
Relative odds of exposure	$= \dfrac{a/c}{b/d}$	$= \dfrac{ad}{bc}$	

You may also come across cohort studies in which (usually) the mortality rate is compared with that expected from the general population. If 'O' is the number of observed deaths and 'E' the expected number of deaths, taking into account the age and sex structure of the exposed group, then the standardised mortality ratio or SMR (= O/E) is also the relative risk in the exposed group compared with the general population. This will be close to the relative risk of exposed to unexposed if exposure is rare in the general population.

The results of a case–control and a cohort study on the effects of smoking are shown in Tables 16.4 and 16.5, respectively. In Table 16.4, note the high prevalence of smoking among the controls. This reflects a) the high prevalence of smoking in men at that time and b) some degree of selection bias in that controls were hospital patients.

The approach to use depends on circumstances. Intervention studies raise ethical issues if subjects will be deliberately exposed to harm, but do ensure

Table 16.4 Case–control study – cigarettes and lung cancer (Doll and Bradford Hill 1952)		
	Cases	**Controls**
Smoker	1350	1296
Non-smoker	7	61
Relative odds (odds ratio) = $\dfrac{1350/7}{1296/61}$ = $\dfrac{1350 \times 61}{1296 \times 7}$ = 9		

Table 16.5 Cohort study – cigarettes and lung cancer				
	Lung cancer deaths	**Person-years at risk**	**Rate/year**	**Annual risk**	**Annual odds**
Cigarette smokers	249	195 754.7	0.001272	0.001271	0.001271
Non-smokers	15	117 187.5	0.000128	0.000128	0.000128

Adapted from Hammond and Horn (1958); rate ratio = 9.938; risk ratio 9.932; odds ratio = 9.930

that the time sequence is met and that intervention and control groups are alike apart from the exposure. Case–control studies allow many possible exposures to be evaluated for one disease, but measurement of past exposure can be difficult and cases may be hard to find unless concentrated – in a hospital, for example. Cohort studies allow the study of many different consequences from a single kind of exposure, but if exposure is rare the cohort may be hard to assemble and adequate follow-up may be a problem.

Relative risk measures association, but we need to know about absolute risks as well, as a large relative increase from a small baseline risk may not be as bad as a small relative increase from a high baseline. Cohort studies do automatically give absolute risk; case–control studies will only do this if designed to sample incident cases from a defined population and time period.

Confounding

The weakness of observational studies is the lack of control over additional factors associated both with exposure and outcome. The result may be a spurious association (or its lack) between two variables, due to their mutual association with a third, confounding variable. For example, the risk of lung cancer is greater in manual workers, but this is largely due to the fact that they are more likely to smoke and smoking is associated with lung cancer.

How can we deal with confounding?

- think of it
- measure/record the presence of the confounder during the study
- allow for it in the analysis.

There is no great mystery – essentially, it is a matter of comparing like with like. The possibilities are:

- stratification
- matching
- statistical modelling.

Stratification

Stratification groups subjects into strata according to predefined characteristics, such as age group, sex or disease severity.

Matching

Matching is an extreme form of stratification where each stratum is often just two subjects; for example, a case–control pair. More than two controls may be chosen per case and the number of controls does not have to be the same for each case. These very fine strata are termed matched sets. Matching is also possible in RCTs.

Statistical modelling

This is the modern approach – heavily dependent on computers. Multiple logistic regression is used for case–control studies and models the odds of being a case, using a multiple regression-like formula:

$$\log(P/(1-P)) = b_0 + b_1x_1 + b_2x_2$$

The right hand side of the equation is called a linear predictor. The variables might be categories; thus it would be allowed to have b_2 sex if variable $x_2 =$ sex was coded as 0 = male, 1 = female. The variable coding for sex is called a dummy or indicator variable. The position is a little more elaborate if there are more than two categories (for example, if race was to be allowed for). In this case, separate dummy variables have to be created for one less than the number of categories constituting the variable.

The odds ratio for variable x_1 adjusted for the other factors is $\exp(b_1)$. Conditional logistic regression is a special variant for matched case–control studies. It is better than a conventional matched analysis because it is possible to match on one or two key variables and model the effects of others.

Poisson regression does the same for cohort studies, this time modelling the disease rate. It is closely linked with Cox regression (used in survival analysis and applied in RCTs and studies of prognosis).

The purpose of stratified and matched analyses is to remove or 'adjust for' the effect of a confounding variable, i.e. the variable(s) defining the strata or matched set. The effect of treatment or exposure is assessed within strata and a single overall 'adjusted' figure is obtained by averaging over the strata.

Modelling effectively does the same – but it is more flexible because you can look for joint effects/interactions very easily. Moreover, matching is expensive (it can be hard to find matches when you are matching on several variables) and unnecessary matching (i.e. on variables that are not confounders) is inefficient, giving wider confidence limits (CL).

Effect modification

Some variables can alter the effect of an exposure; for example, prior immunisation will modify the risk of developing a disease, given exposure. That is, there is an interaction between the effect modifier and the exposure. This is distinct from confounding because the effect will arise even if the exposure is equally distributed across categories of the effect modifier. Again, modelling can detect such effects easily by representing interactions as a product of the variables concerned.

Bias

All studies are potentially subject to bias: a systematic deviation from the truth. Unlike confounding, it cannot be dealt with by statistical analysis. The effect is that 'like is no longer compared with like'.

It can arise when:

- selecting subjects for a study
- allocating them to treatments

- measuring exposure
- attempting follow-up
- analysing and presenting results.

The main protection is to think of the possibility and design it out. Possible strategies include:

- random sampling in surveys
- randomised allocation in intervention studies
- objective rather than subjective end-points
- blinded (masked) assessment and analysis
- high participation
- no missing data
- low drop out (to obtain these final three requires persistence and persuasion).

How much disease is 'due to' a given cause?

The aetiologic fraction (also called population attributable risk) is the proportion of cases of a disease 'due to' a risk factor – it is often expressed as a percentage.

For cohort studies, it can be estimated from the formula:

$$\frac{\text{Total incidence rate in population} - \text{Incidence rate in unexposed}}{\text{Total incidence rate in population}}$$

However, it is not possible to apply this to the Hammond and Horn data in Table 16.5, because the table omits results for other types of tobacco.

For case–control studies, a different formula is used (derived from the one above), which emphasises that the impact on a population depends on the proportion exposed as well as the relative increase in risk:

$$\frac{p(R-1)}{[p(R-1)+1]}$$

Where p = proportion of population exposed to risk factor and R = odds ratio of disease given exposure. For example, if 30% of men smoke ($p = 0.3$), R = 14, aetiologic fraction is 80%. We also see that even if everyone was exposed ($p = 1$) then the proportion of cases still unexplained by the exposure would be about 7%:

$$1 - \{(R-1)R\}$$

Diagnosis

The first problem is what do we mean by 'a case' of a disease? Epidemiologists tend to use one of the following criteria:

- Oddity (in a statistical sense), when a measured value is unusually low or high: if we set an arbitrary cut-off point (e.g. 5th and 95th percentiles), then a constant fraction of the population will be 'ill' and this definition need not bear any relation to symptoms.

- Risk: someone is not considered diseased until they have a 'high' risk of some consequence, e.g. serum uric acid and risk of gout. But where do we draw the line? Cut-off points are not easy to define when risk increases linearly.
- Illness: however, this may exclude many people who could benefit from treatment even though they have no symptoms at present – this is the idea behind screening for cancer, for example.
- Better off: the question now is whether the possibly adverse consequences of treatment outweigh the consequences of not treating the condition. Removing skin moles can leave a scar; we accept this risk when we consider that there is a substantial risk of melanoma.

We infer that a patient has a disease by applying tests. The aim is to distinguish people with the disease from those without. This is an instance of the more general problem of classification.

The basic idea of a diagnostic test is that the likelihood of having the disease is related to the level of some measurable characteristic. Levels of this above a threshold value are termed positive and indicate the presence of disease.

Tests may be pathognomic (i.e. defining the condition) and form a gold standard against which other, surrogate, tests may be compared. Surrogate tests measure a proxy variable for the condition with which we are really concerned – clearly, all screening tests use proxy variables but, in fact, the results of most familiar medical investigations, such as serology for hepatitis B or creatine kinase for myocardial infarction, are surrogates for the actual presence of disease. Surrogate tests are used when they are cheaper, simpler, safer, or more acceptable than pathognomonic tests. These issues are especially important in screening, as it is concerned with the routine search for *asymptomatic* disease.

Where a pathognomic test is hard to define, tests may be evaluated relative to some other surrogate or to the results of a combination of surrogate tests.

Any good diagnostic test will be accurate (or valid) and repeatable.

Accuracy (validity)

For continuous variables, such as blood glucose, we must define the threshold for a positive diagnosis. Given this threshold we can evaluate the test in terms of:

- sensitivity = proportion of diseased who test positive
- specificity = proportion of non-diseased who test negative.

Suppose we want to detect impaired glucose tolerance using venous blood taken two hours after a 75 g oral glucose challenge. The results from a sample

Table 16.6 Sensitivity and specificity		
Blood glucose test result	**Diabetics**	**Non-diabetics**
Positive (> 7.8 mmol/l)	74	9
Negative (≤ 7.8 mmol/l)	26	91
Total	100	100
Sensitivity = proportion of diabetics who test positive = 74/100 = 0.74; specificity = proportion of non-diabetics who test negative = 91/100 = 0.91		

of known diabetics and a sample of non-diabetics might look like those in Table 16.6, using a cut-point of 7.8 mmol/l above which a test is 'positive'; which gives a sensitivity of 74% and specificity of 91%.

Why choose 7.8 mmol/l; why not 6.1 or 8.3? At the best (most discriminating) cut-off point, the difference between sensitivity and (1 – specificity) will be greatest (Table 16.7).

The receiver operating characteristic (ROC) plot is a graphical way to find the optimum and a way of displaying the performance of the test over a range of cut-off points. For detecting impaired glucose tolerance, an ROC plot might look like that in Figure 16.2 (the results of useless, i.e. non-discriminating, tests will lie on the 'line of identity'). Similar analyses can be applied to find the most discriminating cut-off point for ordered categories, such as abnormalities found on cervical cytology.

Summarising test performance
This is measured by the area under the ROC curve (AUC). A useless test gives a value of 0.5, but the data for the impaired glucose tolerance gave an AUC of 0.88 (95% confidence limits 0.82 to 0.94).

Table 16.7 Good and poor discrimination					
a) A test with good discrimination			**b) A test with poor discrimination**		
	Diseased	**Non-diseased**		**Diseased**	**Non-diseased**
Test positive	90	1	Test positive	90	90
Test negative	10	99	Test negative	10	10
Total	100	100	Total	100	100
Sensitivity – (1– specificity) = 0.89			Sensitivity – (1– specificity) = 0		

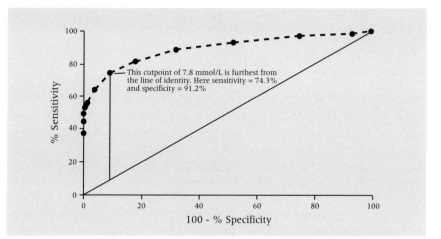

Figure 16.2 The receiver operating characteristic plot – a two-hour postprandial blood glucose ROC plot. Drawn using data taken from Lilienfield and Lilienfield (1980)

Probability of disease given a test result

We need to know the prevalence, p, of the condition in the population tested (the prevalence is likely to be higher in hospital outpatient clinic than in a GP's surgery). The prevalence is the probability prior to the test result of having the disease (hence prior probability).

We must also combine sensitivity and specificity in a single index:

$$\text{The Likelihood ratio for a positive test} = \frac{\text{Sensitivity}}{(1 - \text{Specificity})}$$

The steps are:
- Convert this to prior odds using:

$$\text{odds} = \frac{p}{(1 - p)}$$

that is, the odds of someone chosen 'at random' being diseased.

The Posterior odds are the odds that someone chosen at random is diseased, when they have tested positive:

Posterior odds = Prior odds × likelihood ratio of a positive test

- Convert the odds back to the probability of being diseased, given a positive test result (posterior probability):

$$\text{Probability of disease given a positive test} = \frac{\text{Posterior odds}}{(1 + \text{Posterior odds})}$$

This is also called the (positive) predictive value of a positive test.

We can define the odds of someone who is not being diseased given a negative test too:

Prior odds of health × $\dfrac{\text{Specificity}}{(1 - \text{Sensitivity})}$

Note that the interpretation of the result of a test depends on how common the disease is in the first place ('common things occur commonly'). If prevalence is high, a negative result will not convincingly rule out the diagnosis. Conversely, a positive result will not be overwhelming evidence for the disease if prevalence is low. For example, if the prevalence of disease is 64%, with a test sensitivity of 74.3% and specificity of 91.2%, although the probability of disease given a positive test is 94%, there is still a 33% chance of being diseased if the test result is negative. In practice, for most diseases, the prior probability will not be very high until several investigations have been positive.

The thing to remember is that, in general, high sensitivity rules out the disease, e.g. ERCP for pancreatic cancer: 'if negative, chances are good'. Conversely, high specificity, e.g. liver biopsy for secondary cancer, is not sensitive but 'if positive it is definite'. Sackett *et al.* (1991) use the mnemonic 'SnOUT and SpIN'.

Repeatability

This is the extent to which diagnoses or other measurements agree from occasion to occasion. Typical concerns are the extent to which:

- a single observer's diagnoses are self-consistent (evaluated on different occasions but using the same observer and patients
- the diagnoses made by several observers are mutually consistent (typically evaluated using a panel of observers on a single set of patients).

For interval or ratio scale data, the appropriate index is an intra-class correlation coefficient found using components of variance. This indicates how much of the overall variation in a set of measurements is due to between-patient variation rather than variation in the measurement process itself (disagreement).

For nominal scales, the corresponding index is the κ (kappa) statistic. This is the proportion of cases for whom two observers agree a diagnosis, correcting for the agreement to be expected by chance.

If a panel of observers is used, κ measures the average pair-wise agreement. When only two diagnoses are possible, κ can be shown to be effectively an intra-class correlation and for three or more diagnoses, the overall κ is an average of the κ produced for each category versus the others combined. The idea can be extended to give a κ even when not all the observers in a panel assess every patient (Table 16.8).

In fact, despite their apparent dissimilarity, both κ and intra-class correla-

Table 16.8 Example of κ – two pathologists compared assessments of cervical biopsies (Lambourne and Lederer, 1973)

First observer's opinion	Second observer's opinion Invasive carcinoma	*In situ* carcinoma	Severe dysplasia	Normal/mild dysplasia	Total
Invasive carcinoma	11	0	0	0	11
In situ carcinoma	2	13	0	0	15
Severe dysplasia	0	6	22	1	29
Normal/mild dysplasia	0	1	3	19	23
Total	13	20	25	20	78

Observed proportion of agreements = $(11 + 13 + 22 + 19)/78 = 0.83$

Chance-expected proportion = $(13 \times 11/78 + 20 \times 15/78 + 25 \times 29/78 + 20 \times 23/78)/78 = 0.27$

NB the expected numbers are found as in a χ^2 test as $\dfrac{\text{row total} \times \text{column total}}{\text{grand total}}$

These are added and divided again by the grand total to get the expected proportion of agreement.

$$\kappa = \frac{(\text{Observed proportion} - \text{Expected proportion})}{(1 - \text{Expected proportion})} = \frac{(0.83 - 0.27)}{(1 - 0.27)} = 0.77$$

tion coefficients are instances of a reliability coefficient and can be recast in the general form of:

$$\text{Reliability} = 1 - \frac{(\text{Observed errors}}{\text{Chance-expected errors})}$$

While κ (and intra-class correlations) correct for chance-expected agreement in a given sample of patients and observers, they are affected by the case-mix so that a different sample of patients may give a different κ even if nothing else has changed. This is called the base rate problem and means that κ values are not comparable between different studies unless the proportions of each diagnostic category are similar. For example, suppose we have two observers and three tumour types: 'squamous carcinoma', 'adenocarcinoma' and 'other' and the probabilities of agreement given each tumour type are fixed. A case mix of: 33 squamous, 33 adeno, 34 other gives a κ = 0.55 with standard error = 0.069. However, a case mix of 56 squamous, 29 adeno, 15 other gives a κ = 0.46 with standard error = 0.081, so case-mix affects both κ and its confidence limits.

κ ranges from 1 (indicating perfect agreement) through 0 (indicating agreement no better than by chance) to negative values (indicating disagreement beyond chance expectation). There is no fixed lower limit for κ – unlike an intra-class correlation which ranges from 0 to 1.

What are 'good values'? Landis and Koch (1977) gave the following benchmarks:

- < 0.01   'poor'
- 0.01–0.20   'slight'
- 0.21–0.40   'fair'
- 0.41–0.60   'moderate'
- 0.61–0.80   'substantial'
- 0.8   'almost perfect'.

However, these need to be interpreted relative to what is needed, what it is reasonable to expect and what is possible given the prevalence of each disease category.

In practice, typical values can be disappointingly low. For subtypes of non-small cell lung cancer between-observer κ in one study was only 0.39; similar agreement (between-observer κ of 0.44) has been found on the presence of cholestasis-plugs in liver biopsies, although within-observer κ was 0.766 indicating self-consistency, at least (Theodossi et al. 1980).

A refinement is weighted κ, which takes into account the relative importance of each type of disagreement – for example, if one observer diagnoses 'in situ carcinoma' and the other 'invasive carcinoma', this is much less serious than if one diagnoses 'normal' and the other 'invasive carcinoma'. Weighted κ is most suitable for ordered categories (as in the example above) but even then a generally accepted set of weights for each disagreement may not be feasible. If the data really lie on an interval scale, then it would be better to use an intra-class correlation.

Agreement studies can be improved by:

- standardising measurement conditions
- training to a uniform level of competence
- using objective measurements
- ensuring patients are representative in terms of range and severity of conditions.

Possible applications are to:

- prove comparable performance in assessing patients for RCTs
- demonstrate adequate repeatability for screening programmes
- identify repeatable classifications prior to validation in terms of sensitivity/specificity
- help simplify diagnostic classifications
- identify 'cliques' of observers (whose diagnoses tend to be similar).

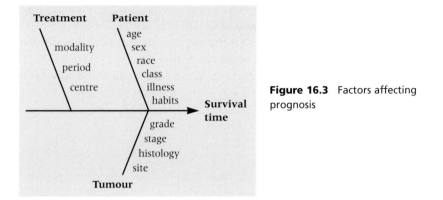

Figure 16.3 Factors affecting prognosis

Prognosis

A prognosis is simply a forecast, or prediction, of the course or outcome of a disease. Characteristics which influence outcome may be summarised in a cause-and-effect diagram, such as Figure 16.3, which summarises factors affecting survival time in cancer.

Typically, prognostic factors, as such, are taken to be properties of the disease state or the patient, but we can extend the concept to include treatment-related factors as well.

Because the forecast is an estimate of what will happen, based on experience with similar individuals in the past, there has to be some uncertainty about the result. For an individual patient, the forecast result may not happen: it can only be 'statistical'. This does not mean that the method used to produce the forecast is wrong, because the forecast only predicts what will happen on average.

A classic form of outcome is death or occurrence of complications. We may extend this by measuring time to the event. This clearly applies to survival from a disease but also applies to time of first occurrence (of a multiple event such as a migraine attack) and survival analysis methods can equally be used for any other non-negative quantity, not necessarily time at all.

Such results can be presented graphically in a survival plot, which displays the proportion of the original subjects remaining alive against time since diagnosis (Figure 16.4).

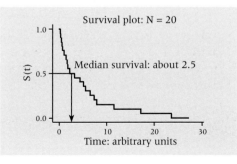

Figure 16.4 Typical survival plot

The y axis in Figure 16.4 indicates $S(t)$ – the proportion of survivors at time t, while t itself is shown on the x axis.

We can use such a plot to read off the median survival or the proportion alive at any given time (the same as the proportion living at least that time). The 'steps' come about because of the way the plot is estimated: survival is constant until someone dies and then it jumps. As the sample size increases, the plot progressively approaches a smooth curve. Modern software packages will construct plots automatically given survival times.

Censoring and withdrawal
One peculiarity of survival data is that survival times may be censored. Imagine 100 patients followed from diagnosis until two years have elapsed. The naïve way to produce a survival plot would be to plot each month the number still alive/100. This survival plot would be straightforward, but suppose a newly diagnosed patient joined the group after 18 months and was still alive six months after diagnosis when follow-up ceased?

We say such an observation is censored, as we know the patient lived at least six months but the exact time survived is unknown. Another way in which censored survival times occur is if patients move away during the two years and are lost to follow-up. Provided this occurs at random we can treat such cases in the same way as if censored due to the end of the study period.

Because of this peculiarity, in practice survival plots are not constructed using the number remaining alive, but are produced indirectly, using the hazard (it is the instantaneous probability of dying).

For each moment in time:

$$\text{Hazard (ht)} = \frac{\text{deaths}}{(\text{Number at risk at time } t)}$$

At each time point, if no patient dies the hazard is 0 and if patients are censored they reduce only the denominator. We then have:

$S(t)$ = Probability of surviving to at least t
      = Probability of surviving each interval to t
      = $(1 - h_1)(1 - h_2)....(1 - h_t)$

This is the Kaplan-Meier estimator of $S(t)$. If values are given rather than a plot, it is a form of life table.

Comparing two or more survival curves is essentially a matter of comparing hazards at each time, effectively by averaging the hazard ratios and calculating a form of χ^2 statistic on the observed number of deaths compared with that expected if the average hazard ratio over time is 1. This is the log-rank test.

Cox regression models the hazard ratio in a multiple regression-like way, allowing for the effect of many variables to be incorporated:

$$\log(\text{RR}) = b_1 x_1 + b_2 x_2 + \dots.$$

As $\exp(b)$ gives the relative risk, if $b > 0$, the corresponding variable increases the risk (shortens survival). If there is more than one variable, exponentiating one coefficient gives the relative risk for that variable, having adjusted for the presence of all the other predictor variables in the equation. Exponentiating the whole linear predictor for a given combination of values gives the total relative risk for that combination.

Forming prognostic groups, validation and discriminatory power

We can form prognostic groups from the distribution of values of the linear predictor. For example, we might define 'good', 'intermediate' and 'poor' prognostic groups by using the lower and upper tertiles of the linear predictor as cut-off points. Note that, since the greater the value of the linear predictor the greater the risk of dying, a high value for the linear predictor is bad news. The linear predictor can now be used directly as a prognostic index. Often, it is a simplified version of the original linear predictor; for example, coefficients may be rounded to the nearest integer.

Once a prognostic index has been constructed for a set of patients, its performance needs to be validated in terms of how well it discriminates between patients 'who do well' and those who do not. In general, a prognostic index will not perform so well on a second or subsequent sets of patients, because it will have been tailored to the original 'training set'. The actual performance can be estimated in a number of ways: one is to have a separate 'validation' set of patients – that is, the prognostic index is cross-validated.

How is the performance of the prognostic index to be measured? One suggestion is to use a rank-based measure of concordance between rankings on the prognostic index and the survival time. The result is a proportion of concordant rankings that can be thought of as a generalisation of the area under an ROC curve.

Case-fatality 'rate' is another measure of outcome – especially useful when the disease is brief, as in plague, cholera or meningitis.

It is defined as:

$$\frac{\text{Number of deaths from a disease in a given period} \times 100\%}{\text{Number of new cases of the disease in the same period}}$$

This can lead to problems when *more* people die of the disease in a given period than develop it. For example, in Trent Region during 1990, 173 women aged 85 years or older died of breast cancer, whereas only 140 women developed the disease. The problem, of course, is that the deaths occur over a period of several years, well after the onset of the disease. It is better to use a different definition, based on the survival curve of patients followed from the point of diagnosis. However, we can also use the survival curve to answer a slightly different question, namely that of 'cure'.

Can we tell if 'cure' is possible? Often, we would like an estimate of the proportion of people who are cured of a disease like cancer – in effect, this is the complement of the case fatality rate mentioned earlier. Some cancers, like those of the pancreas, kill virtually all patients within one or two years, whereas breast cancers have a relatively good survival rate, although even 20 years later the patient may develop a recurrence and die. In general, we cannot be sure that an individual has been cured. We can, however, define a 'statistical cure', applied to a group of people, which can be used as the probability that an individual will be cured.

Demonstration of a statistical cure can be seen graphically (Figure 16.5). If we plot relative survival (i.e. observed/expected) against time, then when the plot becomes constant it can be shown algebraically that, at this point, the annual death rate from all causes is similar to that of a normal population of the same age and sex distribution. We say that this group shows statistical evidence of a cure and the fraction cured is given by the relative survival at the time the plot becomes constant. In the above example, it is about 68% (Figure 16.6).

Such statistical cure seems to have been demonstrated for some cancers (e.g. childhood leukaemia) but not others (e.g. breast). Some difficulties are

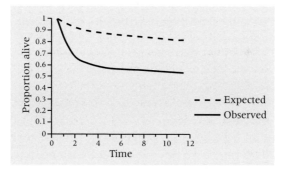

Figure 16.5 Observed and expected survival

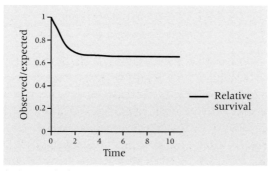

Figure 16.6 Relative survival

that you need a long follow-up to be sure that 'cure' is reached, but, by then, the numbers at risk are relatively small – hence there is in practice a question of sampling error. Also, during a long follow-up, a new treatment may have changed the situation (e.g. penicillin). Moreover, it is important to use the right sort of comparison group: mortality rates should be derived from the same area that has supplied the patients and ideally be comparable with respect to other factors (e.g. smoking, social status and length of residence) that affect death rates. This is hardly ever possible. Lastly, as time goes by, the relative survival curve tends to be weighted towards that of the younger members of the cohort of patients, who by now predominate, giving a falsely optimistic picture of the possibility of cure.

Other forms of outcome

Outcome need not be assessed on an 'all/none' scale or restricted to survival. They may be measurable on an ordinal scale, such as morbidity or pain, or measurable on an interval scale, such as blood pressure, CD4 lymphocyte count or FEV_1. It is important to know, however, whether these are an end in themselves or whether they are a surrogate for some other measure such survival time.

If an indicator like 'quality of life' is measured several times during the course of an illness, it might look like that in Figure 16.7. We can combine quality of life and survival by multiplying each year a patient survives by the quality of life experienced – possibly including a 'discount' factor. The result is the 'quality adjusted life-year' or QALY, often used in determining treatment policies.

Conclusion

The key areas addressed by epidemiology are aetiology, diagnosis and prognosis. These can be applied to and illuminate all branches of medicine – in a sense, epidemiology can be regarded as the true theoretical basis of all medicine, because its concerns are not constrained by accidents of physiology.

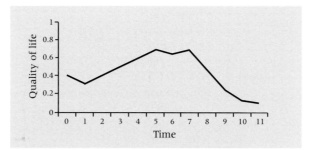

Figure 16.7 Quality of life for a single patient (hypothetical)

References

Doll, R. and Bradford Hill, A.B. (1952) A study of the aetiology of carcinoma of the lung. *BMJ* **ii**, 1271–86

Gardner, M. and Donnan, S. (1977) Life expectancy: variations among regional health authorities. *Popul Trends* **10**, 10–12

Hammond, E.C. and Horn, D. (1958) Smoking and death rates – report on forty-four months of follow-up of 187,783 men. *JAMA* **166**, 1294–308

Hill, A.B. (1965) The environment and disease: association or causation? *Proc R Soc Med* **58**, 295–300

Lambourne, A. and Lederer, H. (1973) Effects of observer variation in population screening for cervical carcinoma. *J Clin Pathol* **26**, 564–9

Landis, J.R. and Koch, G.G. (1977) The measurement of observer agreement for categorical criteria. *Biometrics* **33**, 159–74

Lilienfeld, A.M. and Lilienfeld, D.E. (1980) *Foundations of Epidemiology*, 2nd edn. Oxford: Oxford University Press

Office of National Statistics (E. Purdie, Ed.) (1996) *Guide to Official Statistics* London: HMSO

Sackett, D.L., Haynes, R.B. and Tugwell, P. (1991) *Clinical Epidemiology: A Basic Science for Clinical Measurement*, 2nd edn. Boston: Little, Brown

Theodossi, A., Skene, A.M., Portmann, B. *et al.* (1980) Observer variation in assessment of liver biopsies including analysis by kappa statistics. *Gastroenterology* **79**, 232–41

Further reading

Basic

Fletcher, R.H., Fletcher, S.W. and Wagner, E.H. (1996) *Clinical Epidemiology. The Essentials.* (3rd edn) Baltimore: Williams and Wilkins

Friedman, G.D. (1994) *Primer of Epidemiology*, 3rd edn. New York: McGraw Hill

Kahn, H.A. and Sempos, C.T. (1989) *Statistical Methods in Epidemiology*. Oxford: Oxford University Press

Lilienfeld, D.E. and Stolley, P.D. (1994) *Foundations of Epidemiology*, 3rd edn. Oxford: Oxford University Press

MacMahon, B. and Trichopulos, D. (1996) *Epidemiology. Principles and Methods.* (2nd edn) Boston: Little, Brown

Advanced

Breslow, N.E. and Day, N.E. (1980) *Statistical Methods in Cancer Research, I. The Analysis of Case–Control Studies.* Lyon: International Agency for Research on Cancer

Breslow, N.E. and Day, N.E. (1987) *Statistical Methods in Cancer Research, II. The Design and Analysis of Cohort Studies.* Lyon: International Agency for Research on Cancer

Esteve, J., Benhamou, E. and Raymond, L. (1994) *Statistical Methods in Cancer Research, IV. Descriptive Epidemiology.* Lyon: International Agency for Research on Cancer

Mahesh, K., Parmar, B. and Machin, D. (1995) Survival Analysis. A Practical Approach. Chichester: John Wiley

Morrison, A.S. (1985) *Screening in Chronic Disease*, 2nd edn. Oxford: Oxford University Press

## 17

Ethics, ethics committees, consent and fraud

Richard Kerr-Wilson

Research: any form of avoidance behaviour
Ethics: southernmost county in East Anglia
(Evans 1997)

What have ethics to do with research? What is the purpose of research ethics committees and how do they work? Are they anything more than an annoying, bureaucratic hurdle for the researcher? How and by whom should consent from volunteers be obtained? How effective are these measures in preventing fraud in research? This chapter will attempt to answer these and similar questions that arise in research involving human subjects.

Ethics and research

Ethics can variously be defined as 'rules of conduct', 'the science of morals', 'the science of human duty' or 'the practical application of right and wrong'. Scientific and medical research requires testing a hypothesis against observed facts. The application of ethics suggests that research should be carried out with the minimum of risks to ensure the maximum benefit. In other words, there should be a good chance of finding an answer to the question posed without causing too much harm along the way.

Most people would agree that some form of ethical guidance in research is necessary (Kerr-Wilson 1994). But why have ethics assumed such a prominent position in research in recent years? Is 'the ethics industry' taking itself too seriously (Editorial 1997)? Presumably researchers have not become less ethical in their practice.

Ethical decision making is a dynamic process (Cefalo *et al.* 1994) and is not absolute. It is related in both time and place to the surrounding culture. James Marion Sims' work on vesico-vaginal fistulas was acceptable in nineteenth century Alabama but may not be considered so now (Ojanuga 1993). Even in the 1990s, research approved as ethical in developing countries may be looked on differently in more sophisticated cultures; what is good for The Gambia may be thought unethical in Boston and London. Placebo-controlled research on the use of antiretroviral drugs to prevent perinatal transmission of HIV in Africa has been criticised for not using the best available drugs in affluent countries for comparison (Editorial 1997; Gambia Government/ Medical Research Council Joint Ethical Committee 1998).

An increase in the requirement for ethical review in research is a result of alterations in public perception, greater knowledge of the effects of interventions and changes in technology. Individual choice and autonomy have succeeded the professional paternalism of Sims' day; subjects expect to be asked if they would like to participate in a research project and to be informed of the advantages and disadvantages of doing so. Late effects of investigations in the past, such as x-rays, may not have been apparent at the time of the original research. A radiological study of the bladder during labour was acceptable fifty years ago but, with recognition of the long-term effects of radiation, would not be considered ethical today. New techniques, such as the cloning of mammals by embryo splitting or nuclear replacement, have presented questions that have not arisen before.

Ethical analysis of research

Ethical analysis of research can be approached in three different ways: goal-based, duty-based and rights-based (Foster 1997). The goal-based researcher will consider that ends justify means, that what is achieved for the benefit of mankind as a result of the research justifies the way in which that research is carried out. The outcome is all-important. This is the image of the 'mad scientist' and few researchers would be quite so blind. Most will acknowledge that they have a duty-based aspect owed to their research subjects to cause them minimum harm, although the extent of that duty may be more difficult to define. The third, rights-based, approach considers the research subject first and asks whether the subject is satisfied with the purpose and method of the research. It is this approach that requires adequate information and consent.

It is the responsibility of the research ethics committee to take all these approaches into account when evaluating a research proposal. Each case will be different and the weighting given to each approach will be different. It is the task of the ethics committee to achieve the appropriate balance.

Published guidelines

Many national and international bodies have issued statements on biomedical research involving human subjects. The World Medical Assembly adopted the original Declaration of Helsinki in 1964 and amended it for the fourth time in South Africa in 1996. All biomedical research should be conducted according to the recommendations it contains. Under Part I, Basic Principles, it states that an experimental research protocol should be submitted for review to an independent committee. Section eight of Part I states that: 'Reports of experimentation not in accordance with the principles laid down in this Declaration should not be accepted for publication' (World Medical Assembly 1997).

The Convention on Human Rights and Biomedicine of the Council of Europe adopted in 1996 (Council of Europe 1997) states under Article 16 that research on a person may only be undertaken if:
- there is no alternative

- the risks incurred are not disproportionate to the benefits
- the research has been approved
- the persons undergoing research have been informed of their rights
- the necessary consent has been given and is documented.

The research must not be contrary to the patients' interests; all aspects of the research protocol must be adhered to; results must be recorded truthfully; adequate records maintained and no unjustified claims made for authorship of any publication (General Medical Council 1995a).

All research should be carried out honestly and responsibly (Royal College of Obstetricians and Gynaecologists 1997).

Ethics committees

Before submission of a research protocol to scrutiny by an ethics committee, discussion with fellow researchers or other colleagues may be helpful. This will indicate any ethical inconsistencies or controversies, and save time and possible embarrassment.

A research ethics committee should review all medical research involving human subjects, whether it is being undertaken in hospital, a primary care facility, a research laboratory or the community.

The aim of research ethics committees is to encourage good research. They should weigh the benefits of the research against the risks to the subjects involved (World Medical Assembly 1997). In so doing, they will protect subjects from undue harm and discourage fraud and unsatisfactory results.

Bad research by incompetent researchers is unethical, resulting in wrong conclusions and potential harm to patients. It is the duty of ethics committees, therefore, to review research design and ensure that suitably qualified personnel carry it out, following an appropriate protocol. They need to be satisfied that the aim of the research is reasonable and that the methods proposed are likely to provide an answer to the question posed. There is little point in embarking on research on sickle cell disease in a district of rural England. The number of subjects required to provide a valid conclusion must be reasonable and it should be possible to recruit them within the time suggested. Appropriate technological backup should be available, both laboratory and statistical, with the funds available to support this. Even in West Africa, a study on sickle cell disease may be unethical if the appropriate laboratory facilities are unavailable or unreliable. Subjects should be informed that they are involved in a research project, given details of it and allowed to withdraw at any time without detriment (World Medical Assembly 1997). They should also be advised what will happen when the research is completed. Subjects recruited into a screening study for cancer may feel let down if the investigations, such as ultrasound or serum markers, are no longer available to them when the study finishes.

Research ethics committees are not constituted to review more general ethical problems of medical practice, which should be referred to a more appropriate body.

Local research ethics committees

Local research ethics committees (LRECs) have been in place in each district health authority in the United Kingdom since at least 1992. The body that performs an equivalent function in the United States is the institutional review board (IRB). Guidelines for the working of LRECs have been available from the Royal College of Physicians since 1984 (Royal College of Physicians 1996). More recently, a list of standard operating procedures for LRECs has been published (Bendall 1994).

Members of LRECs are appointed and administered by the employing authority, not the local hospital or Trust. Their decisions should be independent and based on the ethical aspects of the research under consideration; they should not be open to bias, political or financial pressures. If the committee does not have the appropriate expertise among its members to assess the scientific or statistical aspects of a research proposal, then outside advice should be sought.

An LREC should have a constitution and a chairman, who may be either lay or medical. The duration of appointment and the number of members required for a quorum should be specified in the constitution. The recommended size for a committee is around twelve, with representatives of both sexes. There should be at least two lay members and a nurse and a GP should be included. Other suggestions for inclusion are a hospital chaplain, pharmacist and a representative of the junior medical staff.

LRECs have no power of enforcement, but if they are aware of unapproved research being carried out, or of lapses in protocol, the researcher should be advised. If nothing is done, then the LREC should report to their appointing authority and, if necessary, to the appropriate professional organisation. Annual reports from researchers should be required, to ensure that research is completed; incomplete research is unethical, as it is misleading for subjects and may put them at risk unnecessarily.

Multi-centre research ethics committees

LRECs have been criticised for the time they take, their lack of scientific knowledge and, especially where multi-centre trials are concerned, the differences in methods of application and outcome between various committees (Penn and Steer 1995). For these reasons, a system of multi-centre research ethics committees (MRECs) has been set up in the UK (Department of Health 1997). Research is considered multi-centre if it is carried out within five or more LRECs' geographical boundaries. There is one MREC for each region. Each multi-centre protocol is considered by one MREC only. Once MREC approval has been obtained, LRECs in every area involved will be given the opportunity to accept or reject the protocol within a specified time. An LREC can reject a protocol on local grounds, such as being inappropriate for that district or lack of facilities. They are not allowed to amend the protocol, except for purely local reasons that do not affect its integrity, such as providing information for local minorities (Figure 17.1). Unlike LRECs, MRECs are accountable directly to the Secretary of State for Health.

As with LRECs, there has already been concern about the working of the MREC system (Foster 1997; Laurence 1997; Nicholson 1998). However, a little more time is needed to see whether these fears are justified. Meanwhile, review of all research ethics committees within the National Health Service is to be undertaken by the Department of Health in the near future.

Consent

What is 'informed consent' and who should obtain it from research subjects? How does it apply to research in emergencies or involving mentally incapacitated adults?

The doctrine of informed consent is relatively recent and has come about with the shift in attitude from paternalistic concern by the researcher for his

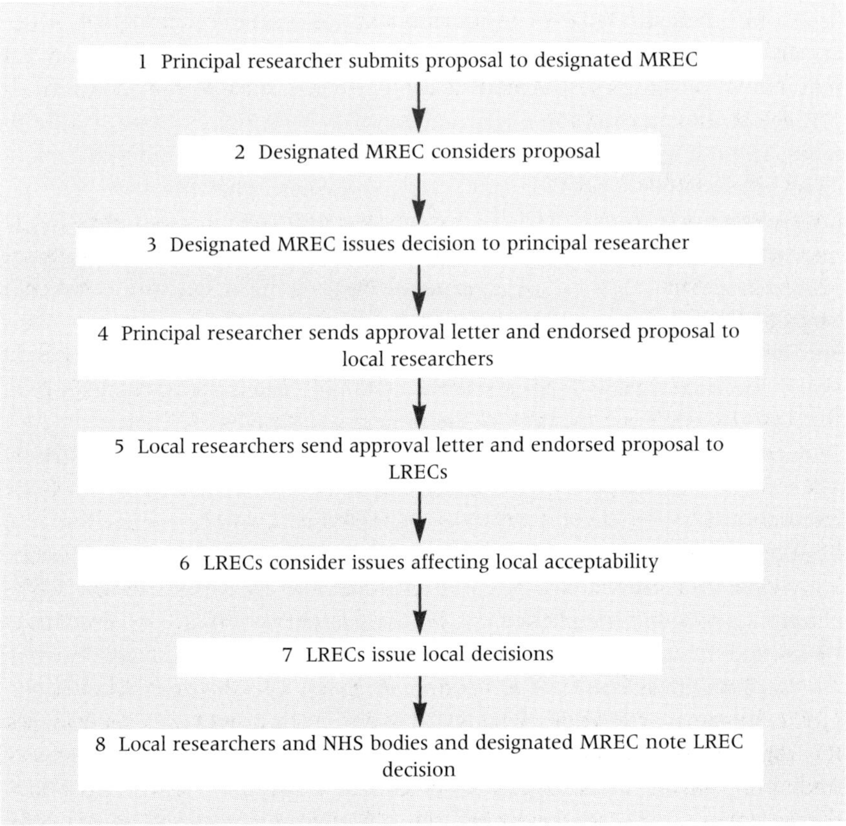

1 Principal researcher submits proposal to designated MREC

↓

2 Designated MREC considers proposal

↓

3 Designated MREC issues decision to principal researcher

↓

4 Principal researcher sends approval letter and endorsed proposal to local researchers

↓

5 Local researchers send approval letter and endorsed proposal to LRECs

↓

6 LRECs consider issues affecting local acceptability

↓

7 LRECs issue local decisions

↓

8 Local researchers and NHS bodies and designated MREC note LREC decision

Figure 17.1 Multi-centre research ethics system flowchart

subject to the self-determination and autonomy of the volunteers themselves (Templeton 1994).

Fully informed consent is an unattainable ideal, since a description of what may occur can never be exhaustive. A complete list of circumstances that may arise during a particular piece of research is not feasible. What is important is that consent is genuine (Nuffield Council on Bioethics 1995). Researchers should communicate the purpose of the research, the procedures and risks involved and the option to withdraw without penalty at any time (Royal College of Physicians 1996; Council of Europe 1997). The information should be provided in written form in a language that is comprehensible to patients, volunteers or relatives. Subjects should be reassured that anonymity will be preserved. If anonymity cannot be guaranteed, subjects must be informed and given the opportunity to withhold their consent to disclosure (General Medical Council 1995b). A third party, such as a research nurse, is probably the best person to provide the information, in order to avoid bias or undue pressure by the researcher. There should be time to assimilate the information and to discuss it with others if requested. An opportunity should be given to talk with the nurse or researcher before asking the volunteer to sign that they have read and understood the information and agree to participate in the research. If all reasonable care is exercised, adequate and genuine consent may be established, even though it can never be 'fully informed' (Nuffield Council on Bioethics 1995).

Special considerations

Special attention to the issue of consent should be given when considering research on children or mentally incapacitated adults (Royal College of Physicians 1996; Council of Europe 1997) and in emergencies (Federal Register 1997). Women who are pregnant, in labour or who are newly delivered also deserve special consideration. They may be consenting for their child as well as themselves, at a time when they are particularly vulnerable (AIMS, the National Childbirth Trust and the Maternity Alliance 1997).

Research on children should only be undertaken if there is no alternative. According to the degree of maturity, the child should be informed of the research and in particular of any risks or discomfort. His or her opinion should be taken into consideration and any refusal or reluctance to participate should be respected. Below the age of 18, in England and Wales, the consent of the parent or guardian should always be sought (Royal College of Physicians 1996).

The Council of Europe Convention on Human Rights and Biomedicine (1997) has devoted a whole Article (17) to the protection of persons who lack the capacity to consent to research. There must be no alternate means of finding the answer to the question being studied and the research must have the potential to produce a real and direct benefit to the individual's health. The necessary authorisation by his or her representative must be given specifically and in writing, and the person concerned must not object. If the research is not for the direct benefit of the person concerned, but in order to obtain a better understanding of the disorder from which that person is suffering, then such research may be authorised providing it entails only minimal risk for the individual. Similarly, in England and Wales, the Law Commission has recommended that non-therapeutic research, which is not intended to benefit the patient directly, may be carried out on patients who lack mental capacity, as long as it is into the condition from which the patient suffers and will not expose the participant to more than negligible risk (Lord Chancellor's Department 1997).

The problem of obtaining consent to research in emergencies has been recognised by the Food and Drug Administration in the United States (Federal Register 1997). Research on human subjects in need of emergency intervention, but who cannot give consent because of their medical condition, is permitted provided the subject is in a life-threatening situation and available treatments are unproven or unsatisfactory. The proposal must be approved by an IRB and the risks associated with the procedure must be reasonable. The subject or his representative must be informed as soon as possible of his inclusion in the study and his option to withdraw.

Research on women in labour has been passed by ethics committees without insisting on informed consent, because of the difficulty in obtaining this at the time (Westgren *et al.* 1998). However, it is recommended that if such research is contemplated information should be provided beforehand, such as in the antenatal clinic, to provide adequate time for explanation and discussion. Women will then be in a better position to give consent, which should be requested at the time of randomisation or treatment (AIMS, the National Childbirth Trust and the Maternity Alliance 1997).

Fraud

No one knows the extent of fraud in research, since it is probably only the most blatant cases that are detected. Few cases appeared until the 1980s in the United States and in Britain, only five had been documented by the end of 1988 (Royal College of Physicians 1991). Fraud involves deliberate deception and may take the form of fabricating data or inventing patients. Forgery of approval by an ethics committee may occur to allow research to take place (Wells and Blunt 1997) or data manipulated to provide the desired answer.

The motive for fraudulent activity may be to enhance academic reputation, for financial gain, as a result of psychiatric illness or merely vanity (Royal College of Physicians 1991). The pressure to 'publish or perish' in academic institutions probably accounts for much of the increase in the number of recent cases. Drug companies often pay a fee for every patient participating in a multi-centre trial, which can result in non-existent patients being entered to receive payment. Two of the best known cases that have come to light lately have been the report in 1994 of the successful relocation of an ectopic pregnancy, when the patient never existed, and the forging of consent forms for patients who never received the drug on trial. In both cases, the doctors concerned were in senior positions in their profession and working in teaching hospitals (Mihill 1997).

The detection and prevention of fraud are not easy. It is less likely to occur when the researcher is junior and is still under supervision. It is more difficult to detect when the researcher is at a senior level in his career and is not supervised. There are two stages at which checks can take place. The first is by the LREC and the second at editorial level, when the research is submitted for publication.

LRECs can help to eliminate fraud by carrying out random audits of protocols submitted. When a proposal is referred to an LREC, researchers are advised that subjects may be contacted in order to audit ethical aspects of the research. The researcher is asked to agree to this, inform the subject that this may occur and be willing to identify patients to the committee for this purpose. A simple questionnaire is then sent to a selected number of patients. They are asked if they are aware that they are taking part in a research project, if they have been given enough information and if they consented to participate (Berry 1997). This process will help to eliminate the use of bogus research subjects, although it will not prevent the fabrication and manipulation of data.

Verification of data can be carried out at editorial level. Instructions to authors should include advice that random requests to review raw data may be made. Submission of an article would either include an agreement to this effect, or be taken as evidence of such an agreement. It would then be up to the researcher to ensure that raw data are kept in a retrievable form and submitted for review if requested. Such a procedure would go some way to preventing the forging of data and help to ensure that research is both accurate and ethical.

Conclusions

A combination of increased awareness by subjects, developments in science and pressure on researchers to publish has resulted in a need for more ethical vigilance in research. All research on human subjects should be reviewed by a research ethics committee to protect not only the subjects but also the researcher. Subjects should be adequately informed about the research before being asked to agree to participate. Safeguards to help prevent fraud should be instituted by research ethics committees and journal editors.

References

AIMS, the National Childbirth Trust and the Maternity Alliance (1997) A charter for ethical research in maternity care. *Bulletin of Medical Ethics* **130**, 8–11

Bendall, C. (1994) *Standard Operating Procedures for Local Research Ethics Committees – Comments and Examples.* London: McKenna and Co.

Berry, J. (1997) Local Research Ethics Committees can audit ethical standards in research. *J Med Ethics* **23**, 379–81

Cefalo, R.C., Berghmans, R.L. and Hall, S.P. (1994) The bioethics of human fetal tissue research and therapy: moral decision making of professionals. *Am J Obstet Gynecol* **170**, 12–19

Council of Europe (1997) 1996 Convention on Human Rights and Biomedicine. *Bulletin of Medical Ethics* **125**, 13–19

Department of Health (1997) *Ethics Committee Review of Multi-centre Research.* Wetherby: Department of Health

Editorial (1997) The ethics industry. *Lancet* **350**, 897

Evans, M. (1997) The essential LREC phrasebook. *Bulletin of Medical Ethics* **125**, 21

Federal Register (1997) Protection of human subjects: informed consent. *Bulletin of Medical Ethics* **132**, 9–11

Foster, C. (1997) Teaching members of research ethics committees: systematic ethical analysis and virtue ethics. *Dispatches* **7**, 1–2 (King's College, London)

Foster, C. (1997) Will LRECs accept MRECs? *Bulletin of Medical Ethics* **133**, 15–16

Gambia Government/Medical Research Council Joint Ethical Committee (1998) Ethical issues facing medical research in developing countries. *Lancet* **351**, 286–7

General Medical Council (1995a) *Good Medical Practice.* London: General Medical Council

General Medical Council (1995b) *Confidentiality.* London: General Medical Council

Kerr-Wilson, R. (1994) Problems with the ethics of medical research. *Br J Hosp Med* **52**, 495–6

Laurence, A.S. (1997) Letter. *Bulletin of Medical Ethics* **133**, 17

Lord Chancellor's Department (1997) *Who Decides? Making Decisions on Behalf of Mentally Incapacitated Adults.* London: HMSO

Mihill, C. (1997) Falsified research 'threat to patients'. *Guardian*, London, 6 November, 5

Nicholson, R.H. (1998) MREC debates continue (Review). *Bulletin of Medical Ethics* **134**, 13–19

Nuffield Council on Bioethics (1995) *Human Tissue: Ethical and Legal Issues*, pp. 44–5. London: Nuffield Council on Bioethics

Ojanuga, D. (1993) The medical ethics of the 'father of gynaecology', Dr J. Marion Sims. *J Med Ethics* **19**, 28–31

Penn, Z.J. and Steer, P.J. (1995) Local research ethics committees: hindrance or help? *Br J Obstet Gynaecol* **102**, 1–2

Royal College of Obstetricians and Gynaecologists (1997) *Ethical Considerations Relating to Good Practice in Obstetrics and Gynaecology.* RCOG Guidelines (Ethics) No. 2. London: Royal College of Obstetricians and Gynaecologists

Royal College of Physicians (1991) *Fraud and Misconduct in Medical Research. Causes, Investigation and Prevention.* London: Royal College of Physicians

Royal College of Physicians (1996) *Guidelines on the Practice of Ethics Committees in Medical Research Involving Human Subjects* (3rd edn). London: Royal College of Physicians

Templeton, A. (1994) 'Informed consent' in: S. Bewley and R.H. Ward (Eds) *Ethics in Obstetrics and Gynaecology*, pp. 287–97. London: RCOG Press

Wells, F. and Blunt, J. (1997) The role of LRECs in the prevention of fraud. Letter. *Bulletin of Medical Ethics* **131**, 2

Westgren, M., Kruger, K., Ek, S. *et al.* (1998) Lactate compared with pH analysis at fetal scalp blood sampling: a prospective randomised study. *Br J Obstet Gynaecol* **105**, 29–33

World Medical Assembly (1997) Declaration of Helsinki (amended 1996). *Bulletin of Medical Ethics* **128**, 8–9

## 18

Supervising and being supervised

David M. Luesley

Background

Good researchers do not know all the right answers but endeavour to ask the right questions. The process of supervising research students should start with this philosophy, to encourage open thinking, critical analysis of data and to define the limits of their generalisations.

This chapter assumes that most, if not all, research supervisors themselves have experience of research. To be effective in research supervision, a supervisor must have both research and supervision skills. Given the above, this chapter purposely omits the other common problems surrounding research such as design, strategy, techniques and methods, reliability and validity. The objectives are those of supervising and being supervised and for the purposes of this chapter relates primarily to higher degrees (PhD, MD and MPhil), although many of the principles equally apply to other research situations, such as undergraduate projects.

Obviously, the needs of each situation differ and an appreciation of this simple fact is essential for all those who wish to supervise research. It follows that the relationship between supervisor and student is not prescribed. All 'research relationships' differ and the differences reflect the project, timescales, levels of academic excellence and, of course, the individual personalities of the parties concerned and how they interact. Nevertheless, there may well be some institutional rules in place that impose a degree of structure on the way research is carried out. This usually relates to regular appraisal or supervision. This is becoming an increasingly important component of funded research, as it is patently a waste of precious resources if the research process founders because of negligent supervision. However, as we shall see later, imposing too rigid a structure may be wasteful in terms of time and may also stifle originality and the development of independent thinking.

Why do people supervise?

Most students expect to have some degree of supervision, but why do established academics wish to supervise others?

Again, this subject largely lies outwith the brief of this chapter, yet it is important to consider it in passing, as it may impinge significantly on the relationship between the supervisor and the student. Academics throughout the

UK regard research as a part of their multidisciplinary brief and, indeed, are to a certain extent assessed on their research output. Supervisors might, therefore, improve their prestige and academic standing by having many research students involved in many, usually related, projects. This might not be to the benefit of individual students in such a programme, unless the supervisor also accords similar high priorities to quality research education and completion of projects. Naturally, this becomes more difficult to achieve as one's work group or team expands and the wise supervisor should always consider the educational implications of research supervision alongside the benefits of high research output for the department. Some universities now impose limits on the number of postgraduate research students for whom any one supervisor may assume responsibility. At present, this does not apply universally. At one extreme, a student may gain considerable and valuable experience through planned and thoughtful supervision from a high profile academic. At the other extreme, a student may be little more than another pair of hands required to fulfil the supervisor's overall goal of running a programme.

How types of project impact on the supervisory process

Projects can generally be divided into exploratory and goal directed phases. In the most simple terms, exploratory means defining the questions. It is involved with approaching new problems or issues about which little is known. The research idea can be less well structured at the outset. In some situations, this phase may occupy most of the time period spent in research. Other types of research or phases within a predefined programme are testing hypotheses (derived from exploratory work), problem-solving (again derived from previous phases) and finally goal-orientated. In most postgraduate medical degrees, research is largely goal-orientated. A problem will have been identified and proposals to address the issue drawn up. The goal is then defined as various steps required to reach that goal.

Most projects will have an initial exploratory component and then a longer goal-orientated component and the needs of each from the supervisor–student relationship differ. The first phase relates to creative thinking and encouraging the student to be confident in developing their own concepts and ideas while the structured phase aims to take the student through the process of planning, data gathering and analysis to test the ideas originally developed. Supervisors should have a firm grasp of the relative components of a project and, with a knowledge of the skills and capabilities of the students, will structure the frequency, content and intensity of the supervision process around the student and the project.

Things to do at the outset

Choosing the right candidate
In real life, students may have little or no influence on who will supervise their research, although they may be able to influence who will not supervise them. Supervisors are either appointed by the research institution or self-selected by virtue of having obtained the necessary resources to undertake a project or programme. Prospective students should aim to work with supervisors who have an established research record in the field of interest and also, although this is not always possible, select a supervisor who has an established record in research supervision.

Similarly, it is vital for research supervisors to select appropriate candidates for research. The selection process will, to a certain extent, be determined by the nature of the project, for instance, if the project requires a significant clinical interface such as counselling and recruiting patients, then a candidate must already have attained a certain level of expertise in this area. Some new skills will obviously need to be brought in and latent talent developed. There is no such thing as the ideal research student, as each individual may posses varying degrees of talent or accomplishment in most of the key areas. These might include:
- the ability to grasp new concepts quickly
- analytical reasoning
- motivation
- perseverance
- organisational skills
- independence
- capability for original thinking
- self-confidence
- previous experience
- can establish good working relationships
  (adapted from Engineering and Physical Sciences Research Council, 1995).

Understandably, any one candidate is unlikely to posses all of these skills and, for these reasons and the difficulty in accurately assessing such attributes, a process of informal interviewing, perhaps on more than one occasion, is useful. This will also allow the potential supervisor to gain some insights into what the potential student wishes to achieve and why they have been motivated to choose you as their supervisor.

Choosing the right project
This may seem simple but, in practice, choosing the right project is both difficult and essential to get right at the outset. In most cases, the student will have selected a particular department because the work conducted within it is of interest to the student. The student should avoid the temptation of taking

on a project just because it is there and has funding. One concept that is always raised with regard to higher degrees is that of originality. That most clinically-orientated projects contain something new is accepted and indeed vital for attaining a higher degree. It is unlikely at the outset, however, that even the most gifted research student can develop flashes of insight and inspiration. It is the author's opinion that part of the research education process is to develop and nurture the intellectual talents of students, in order for them to be able to continue with their own original lines of research.

Prior to embarking on the project, both student and supervisor should go through the plan in some detail to work out rough time frames and what skills may need to be acquired before certain tasks can be taken on and goals achieved. Both should make an attempt to agree at the outset what is reasonable and achievable within the time frames. Both should also recognise that at this preliminary review, the structure of the project should be seen as flexible. The supervisor should make certain that the necessary resources are available for the student to begin, as delays at the outset sap the morale of both. For example, a simple immunohistochemical study, planned as a pilot to a part of the project, may be a reasonable starting point. It introduces the student to new methodology that is both important to the project and a new skill. Results are usually achieved quickly and this is good for the student as it makes them feel well-integrated into the research team and they will have a sense of direction and momentum. If, however, the necessary laboratory space, technical supervision and materials are not available, then a lack of energy can develop which, if not dealt with promptly by the substitution of another equally appropriate task, can lead to feelings of isolation and despair. For most clinicians entering research, there is a major culture shock and supervisors should be well aware of this at the outset.

This initial review may take place over two to three days, some time periods more intense than others. It is useful to use this time as an induction period, introducing the new research student to colleagues with whom interaction will be to the student's long-term benefit. Effort put in by both at this stage sets the scene for the supervision process that follows and also instils in students the notion that, although not necessarily the same type of structured work environment from which they have come (say clinical medicine), research is equally if not more arduous, as time management and self-discipline are new skills.

At the end of this induction phase, it is useful to have some kind of flow diagram or project plan on paper. Microsoft Project™ is a useful package to construct these and it allows back reference in future supervision periods. It also allows the timing of formal supervision periods to be placed well in advance to allow both the student and supervisor to make adequate time and any preparations necessary for these (see below).

Tasks for the supervisor at this stage are:

- setting the ground rules:

   — any rules that apply across the institution
   — any rules that apply in the department
   — health and safety
   — what the supervisor expects from the student
   — what the student can expect from the supervisor, department and
      institution

- determining which skills the candidate has and which will need to be acquired
- deciding how and when they will be acquired
- determining whether the candidate has other skills that can be developed within the scope of the project
- deciding how certain skills will be assessed (plan manuscript writing, departmental presentations)
- inquiring into the student's short- and long-term objectives
- determining the student's interpersonal skills, so that research 'buddies' can be introduced (this is a useful protection against isolation later in the project when the experimental work is at its busiest)
- deciding how the student's project fits in with the rest of the departmental research portfolio.

Dependence to independence

Students should attain independence as the project progresses. One cannot expect students to arrive in any department and be the finished product. The role of the supervisor is to facilitate and effect the transition. The speed at which this occurs varies according to the student, the project and the supervisor. It should be made explicit at the outset that this is one of the key objectives of research training and it should be kept as an agenda item at each formal supervision session. Most clinical research students will have come from an environment where work has been closely supervised and the emphasis has been on clinical training and the acquisition of clinical skills. The weekly timetable is usually fairly structured. Research differs somewhat, as there is an inbuilt desire to allow students to use initiative and take certain risks in the building of a sound intellectual and analytical approach. If each step of the process is outlined in detail by the supervisor with a fixed time-frame, the student will not gain independence and will remain in 'research assistant mode' throughout the training period. To develop independence, the student should be given leeway to develop ideas and test them. They will come to understand the testing process and will also realise for themselves which new skills need to be acquired.

Too much independence is, if anything, worse. Errors in thought and planning occur and eventually the project will grind to a halt. One cannot just give a new research student the protocol and suggest that they go off and recruit 200 patients for an intervention study that could be a part of the project. The problems of recruitment need to be discussed, any background reading fully understood and then suggestions made. Any suggestions that are positive and made by the student should be encouraged, while negative suggestions should be debated and discarded (using constructive criticism), only after the student appreciates why the suggested methodology is bound to fail. This is but one of many positive interactive methods used to teach the experimental and analytical process.

Things that students want

Students expect supervision
Although perhaps stating the obvious, this is one of the most frequent criticisms that students make regarding postgraduate research. There has to be a close adherence to regular and formal supervisory meetings. Reference to previous meetings is vital to ensure that the project is on target and that, if not, problems can be identified early and remedial action taken. For these reasons, the author recommends that both the student and the supervisor make notes at each meeting, if necessary referring back to the 'game plan' and making alterations to future plans as deemed necessary and appropriate within the confines of the project. In at least some medical schools, the DM is not (on paper) a supervised degree. Rather great care is taken to mention only the appointment of an advisor. It is, therefore, important that ground rules for the institution where the work is being undertaken should be established from the start.

Students expect the supervisor to be prepared
Just as the supervisor might expect the student to have any planned work available in a timely fashion, students have the right to expect the supervisor to be prepared for formal supervision periods. This should be both by having read and constructively criticised any prepared work, and in planning the next steps, if necessary by having refreshed their knowledge of that particular area of work.

Supervisors should be available to their research students
Formal supervision sessions apart, problems can and do arise in the intervening period and if the student cannot have access to the supervisor to discuss these problems then inertia might set in until the time of the next supervision. This is precious time lost but, more importantly, morale can suffer. It can be very difficult for busy academics to allow this degree of access, as they are usually involved in many other aspects of academic life. Indeed, the busy and established academic with an international reputation may be the focus for research students, initially for the right reasons, but when it comes down to ease of access, the problems become apparent. A way round this problem is by making one day a week 'open day'. The supervisor knows that this is the time when any of their research students may informally meet and discuss their various projects, while at the same time the students know

that this is the time to make those informal approaches. One must stress, however, that all supervisors and students are individuals who may work in different ways. A mutually agreed method of access should be planned at the outset so that the supervisor and student feel comfortable and secure in the arrangement. One must try to avoid making the student feel that they are imposing on 'valuable' academic time, yet at the same time instil some form of discipline so that time is not overly wasted on trivia.

Students expect an open, friendly and supportive attitude

This is the basis of that underlying bond or relationship that research students have with their supervisors. Constructive criticism requires bipartite and open debate and not a one way didactic process.

Students expect constructive criticism

This is often harder to achieve than first meets the eye. Everyone is sensitive to a degree and, in this situation, the supervisor must not intimidate, yet at the same time they should foster the learning process. Positive feedback and encouragement are required and not a focus on what the supervisor may feel as negative aspects. Encouraging reflective discussion such as 'If you were tackling that problem again, is there anything you would do differently?' followed by 'Why do you feel that would be better?' is beneficial.

Students expect their supervisors to have a good knowledge of the area of research

Often, towards the end of a project, the good student will have greater knowledge in one small area than the supervisor. During the process of arriving at this point, there will and should have been a period where the roles were opposite. At any point, however, the supervisor should always have sufficient knowledge to engage in debate and transference of ideas. This is another fundamental aspect of the research relationship.

Students expect their supervisors to have some responsibility for their futures

Nobody can guarantee employment in what is often a highly competitive field. Nevertheless, the supervisor should, at the very least, guide and support the student in their chosen direction. It is futile to make promises at the outset as a sort of incentive for hard work; the desire to work hard and achieve their goals must come from the students themselves.

Frequency and type of supervision

The supervision process can be divided into three phases:

- The introductory phase, when the supervisor introduces short-term objectives, work to be done and provides detailed feedback and constructive criticism.

- The intermediate phase is more support and guidance than direction. Goals are jointly discussed and planned and any work done by the student is criticised jointly.
- The final phase includes exchanging ideas, although the student makes the decisions regarding the work to be accomplished and the appropriate time frames. More detailed and critical analyses should be provided by the student without any prompting or suggestion.

The primary skill of the supervisor is knowing when the transition between these phases should occur. Formal supervision sessions should be scheduled, at least on a two-monthly basis, but perhaps more frequently in different phases of the project, particularly at the outset.

Conclusions

Meaningful postgraduate research is both difficult, yet immensely rewarding for the student and the supervisor if the goals and objectives are clearly understood at the outset and if both are prepared to work as a team. Students should regard this as a first step in their intellectual evolution toward academic excellence. The experiences during this period, the highs and the lows (of which there will be many) will undoubtedly be a major influence on them and how, ultimately, they will become not only a credible researcher but also an effective supervisor.

Reference

Engineering and Physical Sciences Research Council (1995) *Postgraduate Research: A Guide to Good Supervisory Practice, a Consultative Document.* August 1995. Swindon: Engineering and Physical Sciences Research Council

Further reading

Brown, G. and Atkins, M. (1988) 'Effective research and project supervision' in *Effective Teaching in Higher Education* pp. 115–49. London: Routledge

Cryer, P. (1996) *The Research Student's Guide to Success.* Buckingham: Open University Press

Cryer, P. (1997) *Handling Common Dilemmas in Supervision.* London: Society for Research into Higher Education and Times Higher Educational Supplement

Delamont, S., Atkinson, P. and Parry, O. (1997) *Supervising the PhD. A Guide to Success.* London: Society for Research into Higher Education and Open University Press

Phillips, E.M. and Pugh, D.S. (1994) *How to Get a PhD. A Handbook for Students and Their Supervisors* (2nd edn). Buckingham: Open University Press

Okorocha, E. (1997) *Supervising International Research Students.* London: Society for Research into Higher Education and Times Higher Educational Supplement

Applying for a grant

Katrina M. Wyatt
and Paul W. Dimmock

Introduction

The competition for research money is increasing every year with more researchers chasing ever decreasing sources of funding. The determining factor in deciding whether or not a research project will be funded is the grant proposal. This chapter will cover:

- how to write a research funding proposal
- how to obtain ethical approval for your research
- the types of grants that are available
- the places to look for research funding.

Putting together a grant proposal

It is very important to have thoroughly considered your project and have written a generic proposal *before* a source of funding is identified, as closing dates for research proposals are often only a few weeks after the initial call for grant applications. Remember too, it takes at least eight weeks to receive ethical approval for a project.

The aim of a research proposal is to state the research hypothesis and to demonstrate how the study has been designed to answer this question. It will also need to clearly define who is expected to benefit from the proposed research. Above all, it must sound new and interesting and as if it will increase the corporate knowledge of science, or the health of individuals or the population, if it is to succeed in the competition. In essence, it has to impress and catch the imagination of an august body of highly selected members of the research grant assessment committee.

Below is a list of headings that should comprise every grant proposal:

- title of research
- summary/abstract (often in lay terms if the grant application might be sent to a charitable funding body)
- purpose/aim of investigation (the research question)
- background
- study design
- beneficiaries
- budget and justification of budget
- dissemination

- curriculum vitae of applicants (expertise of applicants and details of the project management team)
- ethics approval.

The background to your proposed research

This should contain a complete, up-to-date and relevant literature search to show the current state of research in the area. This could be presented as a systematic review of the available data. Give details of previous studies to highlight the need for your research. It is very important to include in the background any pilot work or analysis that you have done which supports your proposal. Similarly, if a teaching package or questionnaire has been devised for the project, it could be discussed in the background and then included as an appendix to the proposal.

Study design

This is the most important part of any research proposal. This will prove to the referees that the applicants are capable of delivering on their proposed research project. The study design should include the following:

Setting

You must describe the setting where the research will be carried out, such as in a hospital, GP practice or in the community, and state why this is a suitable place to obtain the patient cohort.

Inclusion/exclusion criteria

These criteria determine the people who will take part in the study and from where they will be recruited. Include a precise profile of these individuals including their age, sex, nature of illness and so on (inclusion criteria). The proposal should also include details of who will not be eligible to take part (exclusion criteria). If the study requires control patients, the proposal should state who they are and from where they will be recruited.

Number of participants

A certain number of patients will be required to answer the research hypothesis. This number should be justified with a statistical power calculation. No grant application will be accepted without the appropriate power calculations; indeed, it would be unethical to conduct any research if it failed to answer the question because of such a basic methodological deficiency.

Intervention

The procedure or intervention which is going to be applied to each person must be described. If the project is comparing more than one treatment, the method of allocation or randomisation of treatment must be outlined. There are very specific techniques required for the randomisation process.

Outcome measures
The outcome measures should be clearly defined. There may be more than one outcome measure (primary and secondary) but the statistical power calculation should be based on the primary outcome of the study.

Data management
Describe how the data will be collected and who it will be analysed by. Will a secondary analysis be carried out by a health economist or statistician?

Time plan
A time plan should be included in the study design with details of the milestones and when the project should have reached them. An example is:
- 0–3 months, training in necessary methodology
- 3–20 months, recruitment and follow-up of patients
- 20–24 months, collating data, writing up project and disseminating the results.

This will clearly show to the referees that the time scale of the research and the project milestones have been thought through in detail.

Feasibility
It is very important to demonstrate that the proposed research is feasible and that the numbers of patients/samples required for the project can be obtained within the given time scale. It will be appropriate to include any details of past success that your department has had in recruitment in similar studies.

The study design should also contain details of how far the research can be generalised, such as what the widespread implications for your research are: for example, the number of people affected by a condition which the investigators are studying and how the research could impact on their lives and on the NHS in terms of practice and health economics.

Beneficiaries of the project
Who will benefit from your proposed research? Sometimes it may be difficult to identify an immediate beneficiary but try to identify the route through which someone will ultimately benefit. It is to be hoped that this will be the patients whose condition you are treating or monitoring, but it could also be the NHS if, for example, your research identified an alternative treatment which reduced the number of nights a patient had to spend in hospital.

The grant budget and the justification for the budget
As the budget is almost certainly going to be cash limited it will need to include what is essential to the project in order for it to be a success. Major items in a budget are often the salaries of the researchers, as well as any secretarial or technical support that the project may require. The salaries should

include likely pay rises, national insurance and superannuation, which the finance department of the hospital or university should be able to provide. Other questions which may need to be addressed in the budget are:

- Does the research require a special piece of equipment or any laboratory consumables?
- Are any associated warranties or running costs required?
- Will the project necessitate any travel between hospitals or to patients' homes?
- Will the results of the project need statistical analysis or health economics analysis? A health economics analysis can be quite expensive but it could add credence to certain projects.

Other aspects of funding to consider are stationery, photocopying, postage, telephone calls and publication costs. It is important to specify the grade of staff required and the length of time they will be employed on the project. Specific quotes for equipment always add credence to a proposal compared with a rough estimate of approximately £X000 for items of equipment. Some funding bodies allow the inclusion of the cost of overheads for the research project. These are usually calculated as a proportion of the overall salary costs.

The research proposal should also include a justification of the proposed budget. One of the things referees are asked to comment on is the financial feasibility and cost-effectiveness of a research project.

Dissemination

The grant proposal will need to include details of how the results of your research are going to be disseminated. For example, conferences and peer-reviewed journals are two obvious means of telling the wider community the results of the study. However, if it is a clinical trial, the NHS Centre for Review and Dissemination at the University of York and the Cochrane Collaboration might be another means of informing the wider medical community. It may also be appropriate to inform the participants of your research about the results, which can be done through consumer groups or specialist magazines. Development of health care guidelines as a consequence of the research is important in clinically-oriented research.

It is very important that the research proposal should demonstrate any collaborative or multidisciplinary approach to the research question, for example if there is a statistician, health economist or social scientist on the project team. It should also demonstrate that the applicants have the local knowledge and expertise to carry out the research and that the study is feasible and cost-effective.

Ethical approval

Although there is no obligation in law for a potential researcher to submit a protocol to an ethics committee for review and approval, it is sensible to get approval by an ethics committee before submission, as their approval may require a modification to the proposal. No institution would allow work to be undertaken by one of its employees, whether involving human or animal subjects, which has not been approved by a ethics committee. The committee is acting as an agent for that institution in determining the cost/benefit of the research, primarily to the individuals who be the subject of the research. The interests of the NHS are secondary to this. Again, while clinical research would usually be aimed at an ultimate therapeutic potential, there are instances of basic medical research being undertaken, the therapeutic potential of which cannot be determined before it is done. Nowadays most funding bodies require a letter of ethical approval to be submitted with the grant proposal.

The role of the local research ethics committee (LREC) is to advise the NHS on the ethical acceptability of research projects which involve human subjects. They are there to ensure that local research is ethically sound, that the rights of patients in the study are maintained and they are protected from harm. In order to gain ethical approval you will need to prove that the project is ethically sound and the research has therapeutic potential. The applicant will also need to prove that the proposed length of the project is reasonable and that any risk to the patient can be justified. It will also need to be shown that the investigator is sufficiently qualified to carry out the procedures.

If you are going to obtain informed consent from the patient (and almost all studies will require it if patients are involved) then you will need to include a consent form and a patient information sheet with the approval form from the ethics committee. The patient information sheet is very important; often ethical approval is withheld because of problems with this. It must be written in clear and simple terms at an appropriate reading age, tell the patient exactly what procedures they are going to undergo and what being part of the study entails. It will also need a statement saying that they can leave the study at any time and their care will not be affected. For multi-centre trials, ethical evaluation will be divided between a multi-centre research ethics committee (MREC) and LRECs. The LRECs will have responsibility for decisions on local practical issues concerning the research. Overall ethical approval for a multi-centre research project should be sought through one of the regional multi-centre ethics committees which, once obtained, will enable rapid local approval to be given. Chapter 17 considers the ethics of research and consent in detail.

Rejection of a grant proposal

Be prepared to re-submit your proposal to different funding bodies. If the grant is rejected, ask for feedback from the funding body to which it was sent, some will automatically provide written comments from the referees, others will give informal feedback over the phone. Also ask for feedback on the proposal from colleagues who already hold a grant, if this has not been done at the outset. Any new researcher (perhaps any researcher) should seek the views of colleagues before the original submission.

Types of grant available

- fellowships (a personal award made to an individual for their salary and some associated research costs)
- project grants (a cash-limited award to enable a research question to be answered)
- programme grants (ambitious award to enable a series of related research questions to be answered)
- travel and exchange (funding to attend an appropriate conference or funding to permit a sabbatical in another research institution)
- equipment and laboratories
- conference/workshop (funding for a conference or workshop to take place)
- industrial collaboration (this can be directly funded or jointly funded between industry and a research council).

Not all funding bodies provide all the above types of grants. Ultimately, the research proposal will determine which is the most appropriate type of grant to apply for. However, for people who are beginning a research project, applying for either a fellowship or a project grant could be a suitable starting point. It will strengthen the application for both these types of grant if they are applied for in conjunction with an experienced colleague who has an academic or research track record.

A fellowship is primarily to fund your salary, thus enabling you to undertake your research project. A lot of fellowships are called training fellowships because they do not expect the researcher to have much, if any, research experience. A fellowship award will also fund some consumables and travel, but in general it will not fund anyone else's salary. If the project requires additional technical or secretarial support, then you probably ought to apply for a project grant. Although project grants are cash limited, they will fund all aspects of your project. It could be that the project determines which of the two is the most appropriate for the proposed research.

Funding bodies

Charities
The Association of Medical Research Charities represents 88 charities which fund medical research. They publish a booklet which details the types of grant they offer and the amount they are prepared to fund.

Research councils
The research councils such as the Medical Research Council and the Biotechnology and Biological Sciences Research Council offer all the types of grants mentioned earlier.

The NHS Executive

The NHS supports research at a local and national level. Locally-organised research schemes offer project grants, clinical and non-clinical training fellowships and one-off equipment grants to researchers within the local health authority. From time to time applications are invited for support for research related to national priorities and these tend to appear in national newspapers such as *The Guardian*. Similarly, the Department of Health occasionally has a call for proposals in a particular area of health care.

Industry

Some pharmaceutical and technology companies offer travel bursaries and small project grants. These tend to be advertised in medical journals such as the *British Medical Journal* or the *Lancet*.

Wellcome Trust

The aim of the Wellcome Trust is to promote research in medicine, related basic sciences and other subjects which have the potential for improving human welfare. They offer all the types of grants mentioned earlier.

Joseph Rowntree Foundation

The Joseph Rowntree Foundation funds a programme of research and development in the fields of housing, community care and social policy. There are no formal application forms. They suggest sending in an outline proposal (one page) and the project suitability will be assessed and if relevant a full application will be invited.

The National Lottery

The National Lottery does fund some medical research; however, it will only accept one application per medical charity and so your hospital or university will only be allowed to put forward one proposal. Programmes will not be funded if the National Lottery believes that another body such as the NHS or MRC should fund them.

European Union

The key principle underlying the research funded by the European Union (EU) is the fostering of co-operation between member states (the principle of subsidiarity means that the EU will not support research for an individual state). The research must include at least three member states (more details can be found on the EU website, given at the end of the chapter). It strengthens the proposal if the research aims to improve the industrial competitiveness of the EU. The applicant will need to show that the success of the project requires the involvement of all the EU countries collaborating in the research project. Usually, collaboration with countries less advanced in research is considered desirable.

Where to apply

When considering where to apply for funds you will need to consider the level of funding, the type of grant being offered and the length of time that the grant will run for. Another point to be aware of is how much intellectual freedom you will have; for example, if it is a drug trial funded by the drug company, ensure that you have the right to publish the results.

Lastly, some funding bodies such as the Medical Research Council offer a career pathway such that if you are awarded a clinical training fellowship you would then be encouraged to apply for a clinical scientist fellowship and so on up to a professorship.

Why grants are turned down

Grants are turned down for various reasons, such as:

- unoriginal research proposal
- unrealistic project
- not financially viable
- too expensive
- case for funding not set in context
- unsuitability of project for type of grant
- insufficient expertise of applicant
- missed deadline.

Although competition is increasing and funds are dwindling there is research money to be awarded. Probably, the single most important factor in determining whether or not your grant is successful is whether the referees and assessing committee find your proposal interesting.

Useful addresses and websites

Medical Research Council

20 Park Crescent, London W1N 4AL. Tel. 0171 636 5422; fax. 0171 436 6179
Internet: http://www.mrc.ac.uk

Association of Medical Research Charities

29–35 Farringdon Road, London EC1M 3JB. Tel. 0171 404 6454
Internet http://www.amrc.org.uk

Charities Aid Foundation

King's Hill, West Malling, Kent ME19 4TA. Tel. 01732 520000
Publishes *The Directory of Grant Making Trusts.*
Internet http://www.charitynet.org.uk

NHS Health Technology Assessment

Lynn Kerridge, National Co-ordinating Centre for Health Technology Assessment

Tel. 01962 863511; fax. 01962 877425
Internet: http://www.soton.ac.uk/~hta/advert.htm

The UK National Lottery
St Vincent House, 30 Orange Street, London WC2H 7HH. Tel. 0171 747 5299
Internet: http://www.nlcb.org.uk

European Union – Fifth RTD Framework Programme 1998–2002
Internet http://www.cordis.lu
Fax. for Biomedicine and Health (BIOMED) 00322 295 5365

Engineering and Physical Sciences Research Council (EPSRC)
Polaris House, North Star Avenue, Swindon SN2 1EZ. Tel. 01793 444100
Internet http://www.epsrc.ac.uk

Economic and Social Research Council (ESRC)
Polaris House, North Star Avenue, Swindon SN2 1UJ. Tel. 01793 413000
Internet http://www.esrc.ac.uk

Biotechnology and Biological Sciences Research Council (BBSRC)
Polaris House, North Star Avenue, Swindon SN2 1UH. Tel. 01793 413200
Internet http://www.bbsrc.ac.uk

Wellcome Trust, Grants Section
183 Euston Road, London NW1 2BE. Tel. 0171 611 888; fax. 0171 611 8545
Internet http://www.wellcome.ac.uk

Industry – Association of British Pharmaceutical Industry (ABPI)
12 Whitehall, London SW1A 2DY. Tel. 0171 930 3477
Internet http://www.abpi.org.uk

WellBeing and Royal College of Obstetricians and Gynaecologists
27 Sussex Place, Regent's Park, London NW1 4SP. Tel. 0171 262 5337
Internet http://www.rcog.org.uk

Joseph Rowntree Foundation
The Homestead, 40 Water End, York YO3 6LP. Tel. 01904 629241

20

Communicating research: working with the media

David A. Grimes

Introduction

Two centuries ago, Benjamin Waterhouse, a US physician, learned of William Jenner's discovery of the smallpox vaccination. Waterhouse immediately recognised the public health importance of communicating this breakthrough to the public. 'As the ordinary mode of communicating even medical discoveries in this country is by newspapers, I drew up the following account of the Cow Pox, which was printed in the *Columbian Centinal* (a semi-weekly newspaper published in Boston) March 12, 1799' (Altman 1976). While the medium may have changed (to television), the message remains the same: the media are the public's principal source of medical information. How, then, can researchers capitalise on this fact?

Often unknowingly, researchers routinely address two audiences: the scientific community and the broader lay public. Few researchers today have the latter audience in mind as they conduct and report their work. Nevertheless, reporting of medical research in the print and broadcast media is a huge, and hugely important, enterprise. Research is of no use unless it is communicated. This chapter will describe the often tense relationship between researchers and the media and will offer some pragmatic (although unscientific) suggestions for developing a symbiotic relationship.

The importance of researchers for the media

The lay public and its media have a long-standing fascination with health. Its relevance to the individual is obvious. Interest in medical research is also keen. This stems not only from the hope for important breakthroughs, such as prevention of vertical transmission of AIDS, but also from a proprietary interest: in many developed countries taxpayers foot the bill for much biomedical research (Altman 1976). The public has a legitimate interest in learning the results of the research they have been collectively funding.

Highly visible medical journals provide a rich source of stories for journalists. In the UK, broadsheet newspapers such as the *Telegraph*, the *Guardian*, the *Independent*, the *Observer* and the *Times* all have at least one journalist who scans every issue of the *Lancet* and the *British Medical Journal* for stories. They expect to find at least one story per week from these two sources (Entwistle 1995). In the US, health reporters for major metropolitan newspapers and the wire news services follow closely the press releases of the *Journal of the American Medical Association* and the *New England Journal of Medicine*. The latter casts a long shadow and is even the most widely cited journal in Dutch newspapers (van Trigt *et al.* 1994). The competition for hot stories is keen and journals have had to set embargoes on news coverage to avoid rushed stories by journalists trying to beat the competition into print.

Journalists rely heavily on a handful of journals for two main reasons. First, they believe (often incorrectly) that the most important research appears in these journals. Secondly, they trust (often inappropriately) that the peer-review process guarantees valid science (van Trigt *et al.* 1994) The lead article in the 15 January, 1981, issue of the *New England Journal of Medicine* (Darsee and Heymsfield 1981) was later retracted as fraudulent (Heymsfield and Glenn 1983) and is a famous example of peer-review fallibility. Regrettably, negative reports that are unable to confirm 'breakthroughs' are not newsworthy. Corrections or retractions of flawed research generally get no attention in the media. Only scientific fraud seems to be newsworthy. Dissemination of poor science, whether due to misconduct or innocent error, has the same net effect: misleading the public.

The importance of the media for researchers

While researchers are clearly important to the media, the media are similarly important to the scientific community. As noted above, the media are an extension of health care providers in conveying health information. Numerous surveys in developed countries testify to this fact. Television is especially important. The average US citizen watches 7.4 hours of television a day. In the US, the likelihood of reading a newspaper is related to income and the likelihood of watching television is inversely related (Dan 1990). The lower the socio-economic class, the greater is the importance of broadcast media. Given this huge exposure of the public to broadcast and print media, researchers have an ethical obligation to communicate through them (Altman 1976). While television coverage is usually simplistic, newspaper and magazine coverage of health issues often presumes a rudimentary understanding of science. In contrast, large proportions of the public have little knowledge of science and its methods. The recurring reports of sightings of Bigfoot, Elvis Presley and extraterrestrials in tabloids provides indirect evidence of this scientific naïveté.

The media also play a key role in conveying medical information to researchers and clinicians. Like the general public, researchers read newspapers, watch television and listen to the radio. The Internet is likely to play an increasingly important role as its use expands. It is not only the public who learn of research through the lay media; surveys of US physicians suggest that 60–89% sometimes learn of new scientific developments from newspapers (Phillips *et al.* 1991). One report quantified the impact of newspaper coverage of research published in the *New England Journal of Medicine* (Phillips *et al.*

1991). Articles covered in the *New York Times* received a disproportionate number of scientific citations when compared with 'control' articles that were published in the same journal but that did not have newspaper coverage. For example, in the first year after publicity in the *New York Times*, these research articles had 73% more citations by other authors in the *Science Citation Index* than did control articles without newspaper coverage. In contrast, when the *New York Times* shut down due to a strike, this effect disappeared. This natural experiment suggests that newspaper coverage itself, and not 'earmarking' of high-quality research, was responsible for the higher scientific visibility.

'Throwaway' periodicals (free publications supported by advertising) also contribute to the continuing education of clinicians. These have greater readership than do peer-reviewed journals, which are obtainable only by subscription or through organisation memberships. US periodicals such as *Ob/Gyn News* (a free newspaper) and *Contemporary Ob/Gyn* (a glossy magazine) enjoy wider readership than do *Obstetrics and Gynecology* or the *American Journal of Obstetrics and Gynecology*. Hence, researchers who want to communicate with rank-and-file obstetricians and gynaecologists may target these publications. For example, presenting research at certain professional meetings carries a high likelihood of coverage by *Ob/Gyn News*, which sends reporters to meetings. Similarly, after an article appears in a peer-review journal, some researchers write a lighter, derivative piece of about 1500 words for *Contemporary Ob/Gyn*. The magazine provides attractive graphics, an appealing layout and a loyal readership.

The media also serve an important role in research: recruiting participants. Researchers often use newspapers to advertise research protocols. These announcements reach a wider audience than do notices posted on bulletin boards in a medical centre. Drawing research participants from a broader population can improve the external validity (ability to generalise) of a study. A disadvantage of this approach is that readers of newspapers tend to be better educated than those who do not read newspapers. Hence, lower socio-economic strata may be under-represented among participants recruited by this means.

Researchers' reluctance to work with the media

Despite the influence of the media, powerful disincentives deter many researchers from collaborating. First, many scholars view colleagues who work with the press as self-aggrandising. Media attention may feed their need for visibility or simply be a ploy to attract patients to their clinical practices. Co-operating with the press, to some lofty academicians, is tantamount to getting in bed with the devil.

Secondly, a corollary of Murphy's law seems to govern interactions with the media: they have an uncanny knack of calling at inopportune times. Their urgent inquiries often correspond with urgent medical business already in progress. The reporter cannot wait; his or her editor needs the material now.

They want to send over a film crew to tape a commentary when you are scheduled to be in the operating theatre.

Thirdly, many researchers fear the loss of control of their work in the rough-and-tumble world of lay media. Highly technical research is prone to misinterpretation by lay reporters and, unlike professional journals, lay publications do not offer researchers the reassurance of galley proofs. Some publications do, however, have an editorial assistant call back to 'fact check' and confirm quotations for attribution.

A fourth problem is bias. Publication bias is a major problem in professional literature: positive studies are more likely to get submitted and published than are negative studies. Thus, readers draw conclusions (often incorrect) from a skewed and incomplete database.

Publication bias is even more acute in the lay media. Media tend to report positive studies and ignore the rest (Proudfoot and Proudfoot 1981; Koren and Klein 1991). A *Wall Street Journal* reporter commented that this was not really a bias against negative studies but rather a bias in favour of positive studies (Bishop 1992). A newspaper reporter admitted that 'selling a study that shows no results to an editor who doesn't understand science can sometimes be a tough task' (Neus 1992).

The net effect is the same: systematic distortion of the evidence. One example is the putative relationship between alcohol consumption and breast cancer (Houn *et al.* 1995). Of 58 scientific publications during a specified interval, only 19% were mentioned by the press. Indeed, 77% of the lay press stories cited three scientific publications. No reporters referred to review articles on this topic. Stated alternatively, reporters ignored the bulk of scientific knowledge on this question. Another example with harmful public health impact has been print and broadcast coverage of the putative relationship between oral contraceptives and breast cancer (Grimes 1990). In contrast, how many women have been made aware of the protection given by the oral contraceptive pill against ovarian cancer?

Bias can be even more overt. Reporters and editors may slant stories intentionally. An interesting variant of this is the balanced story with an inflammatory headline, written by someone else at the newspaper. Since many casual readers get no further than the day's headlines, the damage may be done with few words, such as 'Killer pill!'

Severe time limitations from reporting deadlines often produce unbalanced coverage. Reporters may have the interest but not the time to do background reading (Entwistle 1995). Their story may be due in 45 minutes. Research operates at a different pace. Few reporters will ask about or describe the rigour of research methods (Houn *et al.* 1995). None the less, this context is necessary to avoid the over-interpretation of results.

Limitations in coverage (column space in print and time in broadcast media) can make adequate exposition impossible. Trying to condense complex research topics into a 60-second spot on the evening news is difficult

(Dan 1990). Important information may be lost in the compression. 'Summarising a research paper in a few hundred words is hard enough, but having to summarise comments on it as well, with no extra word allowance, is even harder' (Entwistle 1995).

Finally, reporters assigned to cover medical research may not be knowledgeable in the subject area. Their editors may assign them stories on rotation. Thus, a common tendency is to look for the 'quick hit'. The measured pace of science is incompatible with this hit-and-run approach to communication.

Why bother?

Given these hurdles, why should responsible researchers get involved in communicating their work (and commenting on that of others) to the public? Consider the alternative. 'As long as the responsible leaders keep silent, the quacks and charlatans will fill the vacuum' (Altman 1976). Indeed, working with the press is an affirmative duty of responsible scientists: '... it is honourable to speak out to the press, to provide facts, to correct errors, and to give reasonable testimony on controversial issues ... If you do not meet your responsibilities, you will continue to subject yourselves to a selecting-out process' (Altman 1976). Having poorly qualified persons pontificating on medical research is painful to all reputable scientists. It is also largely preventable.

Getting started

Accept the rushed schedules of reporters
The inconvenience of disrupting your schedule at short notice will often pay big dividends. Thirty seconds of coverage on a network news broadcast may reach tens of millions of viewers. A ten-minute interview with a women's magazine reporter may reach more people than a physician could counsel in a hundred lifetimes of professional practice. The media become medical education extenders on a massive scale, in contrast to the usual one-to-one consultation.

Expect inaccuracies
Without question, the media will occasionally misquote or misinterpret a researcher, either due to an innocent error or to an intentional bias. This happens to all public figures and is part of the price one has to pay for working in this arena. Nevertheless, the benefits of conveying responsible, important health information to vast numbers of consumers far outweigh the risk of occasional glitches.

Volunteer to help
Newspapers, radio stations and television stations are often eager to find physicians and scientists willing to provide them stories or to comment on others. To have a pool of knowledgeable commentators who can comment on

research in women's health makes a reporter's job easier, especially given their tight schedules. Simply call the news room, identify yourself and express your interest. This can provide excellent training in media for researchers and physicians.

For the novice, many medical institutions sponsor courses or seminars on how to work with the media. These media training exercises may involve not only internal staff but also journalists from the community. A comfortable way to make the initial plunge is with an escort: the media office of your institution. Many hospitals, medical schools and research organisations have press offices and public-relations staff to guide researchers through the experience. These colleagues appreciate learning of new research of general interest, so that they can develop press releases and schedule interviews as appropriate. They understand well that favourable media attention generates philanthropy and more research support: success begets success. In addition, they often know the local press well and can anticipate likely questions and interview styles. They often sit in during interviews and can help facilitate the exchange.

Tips for working with the media
Few researchers have had formal media training. Hence, a few suggestions (Grimes 1990) may make interviews more effective.

Control the interview
Plan in advance what two or three points you want to convey. Regardless of what questions are posed, doggedly steer the discussion back to cover your key points. While this approach strikes the uninitiated as evasive, experience has shown the importance of sticking to a predetermined set of informational bullets. You can only transmit two or three messages in an interview; you should determine them, not the reporter.

Provide historical context
Medical practices or health care policy decisions should rarely be based on a single study, no matter how large or how well done. Reporters unfamiliar with the field often view a single study in isolation. New studies need to be viewed in the light of existing knowledge. When commenting on your own research (or that of others) provide the reporter with a 'discussion section' even if they only request a 'results section'. This involves discussing the strengths, weaknesses and potential biases in the research.

Explain the known risks and benefits
If a reporter inquires about the potential association between alcohol consumption and breast cancer, describe the protection moderate drinking affords against heart disease. Researchers need to provide the balance, since few reporters will have the requisite knowledge for balanced reporting. 'Faced with a strict word limit, journalists said that they found it impossible to

include all the caveats and qualifying statements that are often found in research reports without killing their story' (Entwistle 1995). Unless researchers volunteer these caveats, oversimplification will occur by default.

Keep comments brief for broadcast media

Practice speaking in '20-second sound bites'. Because of the severe time limitations in broadcast media, lengthy responses are often unusable or are severely edited. Keep your comments crisp and concise; sentences of 20 words or less are easier for listeners and viewers than are longer expositions.

Use simple language

Medical jargon ('medspeak' or 'medicalese') may be lost on the lay public (Friedman and Pennisi 1996). Use plain English equivalents, such as 'cancer of the inside lining of the uterus', not 'endometrial cancer'. Aim for English understandable by a child of 12 to 14 years of age.

Give examples

'If 100 women use the Yuzpe regimen for emergency contraception after unprotected intercourse, about two will find themselves pregnant at the end of the month. Without the treatment, about eight will get pregnant.' This is much easier to understand than saying that the Yuzpe regimen 'prevents about 75% of pregnancies that would have occurred without treatment'. While true, the lay public may infer (incorrectly) that 25% of women will find themselves pregnant at the end of the month, not 2%.

Conclusion

'Doctor' does not mean 'healer'. The word derives from the Latin verb docere, to teach. Yet 'doctor' is not a misnomer: only through teaching and communicating do we become effective healers. Physicians traditionally focus on the individual patient. However, our ethical and moral responsibility extends to the broader public. Communicating through print and broadcast media is a natural extension of our obligation to the individual. Working with the media can both improve public health and increase scientific literacy. If we fulfil this public responsibility, everyone benefits. If we default, the opposite is true as well. What gets communicated to the public should be not only newsworthy but also worthy news.

References

Altman, L.K. (1976) Communicating with the public: a physician's responsibility. *Bulletin of the American College of Physicians* **17**, 6–8

Bishop J.E. (1992) Reporting negative studies in the mass media. *Journal of the American Medical Association* **267**, 930

Dan, B.B. (1990) 'Communicating public-health information through the mass media' in: J.C. Bailar III, M. Angell, S. Boots *et al.* (Eds) *Ethics and Policy in Scientific Publication*, pp. 247–9. Bethesda, Maryland: Council of Biology Editors

Darsee, J.R. and Heymsfield, S.B. (1981) Decreased myocardial taurine levels and hypertaurinuria in a kindred with mitral-valve prolapse and congestive cardiomyopathy. *New Engl J Med* **304**, 129–35

Entwistle, V. (1995) Reporting research in medical journals and newspapers. *BMJ* **310**, 920–3

Friedman, E.A. and Pennisi, J.A. (1996) Eschew obfuscation. *Obstet Gynecol* **87**, 795–6

Grimes, D.A. (1990) 'Breast cancer, the pill and the press' in: R.D. Mann (Ed.) *Oral Contraceptives and Breast Cancer*, pp 309–22. Carnforth: Parthenon

Heymsfield, S.B. and Glenn, J.F. (1983) Retraction. Darsee, J.R., Heymsfield, S.B. Decreased myocardial taurine levels and hypertaurinuria in a kindred with mitral-valve prolapse and congestive cardiomyopathy *New Engl J Med* 1981; **304**, 129–35. *New Engl J Med* **308**, 1400

Houn, F., Bober, M.A., Huerta, E.E., Hursting, S.D., Lemon, S. and Weed, D.L. (1995) The association between alcohol and breast cancer: popular press coverage of research. *Am J Public Health* **85**, 1082–6

Koren, G. and Klein, N. (1991) Bias against negative studies in newspaper reports of medical research. *JAMA* **266**, 1824–6

Neus, E. (1992) Reporting negative studies in the mass media. *JAMA* **267**, 930

Phillips, D.P., Kanter, E.J., Bednarczyk, B. and Tastad, P.L. (1991) Importance of the lay press in the transmission of medical knowledge to the scientific community *New Engl J Med* **325**, 1180–3

Proudfoot, A.D. and Proudfoot, J. (1981) Medical reporting in the lay press. *Med J Aust* **1**, 8–9

van Trigt, A.M., de Jong-van den Berg, L.T.W., Haaijer-Ruskamp, F.M., Willems, J. and Tromp, T.F.J. (1994) Journalists and their information sources of ideas and information on medicines. *Soc Sci Med* **38**, 637–43

21

Presenting a paper

Andrew Hextall
and Linda Cardozo

Introduction

Attending a scientific meeting brings with it many benefits and, for some, represents a highlight of the academic year. These include academic aspects such as learning new information, developing new ideas, networking, establishing research with other centres and keeping abreast of the politics of the specialty. There may be social aspects, the chance to visit a new city or even a new country, enjoy the local hospitality, meet up with old friends and sometimes make new ones. It is also considered prestigious to have a paper accepted, especially if it is for a podium presentation at a major conference. However, for the trip to be particularly successful, it is important that the presentation goes well. The following chapter gives some guidelines that will help make this outcome more likely.

Preparation

Even though a project may have been under way for many months or even years, it is often difficult to avoid waiting until the last minute to prepare for an oral presentation. It is vital that adequate time is spent planning your approach and making numerous revisions if necessary. Before you begin, ask yourself the following questions:

- What is the main message of my presentation?
- How much time do I have allocated for my talk?
- Who is likely to be in the audience?

The abstract submitted to the meeting will provide a useful starting point and it is important to stick closely to the methods, results and conclusions included in it. Further help will probably come from the conference organisers, who will inform you how long you are expected to speak for and the amount of time allocated for questions. It is likely that you will know if the audience will be professors of obstetrics and gynaecology, specialists with an interest in your subject, generalists with some background knowledge or a mixture of health care professionals, some of whom may be non-medical and for whom the concept about which you are talking is entirely new. Try to pitch your talk at the right level, so that there is something for everyone in a mixed audience, without losing the main points of focus.

Visual aids

Slides, videos and props should be considered complementary to your oral presentation and provide a structured framework for both yourself and your audience. At almost every meeting most people use 35 mm slides but computer-generated presentations, now available with new software packages (see Chapter 3) are becoming more popular. Do not try out a new technique for the first time at an international meeting. The facilities available will also be outlined by the conference organisers, but if you are in doubt or have a special requirement, telephone the conference secretariat or chairman of the meeting as soon as possible to make sure you get your preparation right.

It is really important to mix the text slides with pictures, graphs and tables to maintain everyone's interest. There are several rules to follow when making slides which will improve your presentation tremendously (Table 21.1). The temptation is always to use too much text to ensure that you do not forget to say anything crucial. This results in too small a font size being used, with too many words for the audience to digest at the same time as listening to what you have to say. Always try to design your slides so that they can be easily seen and read by people at the back of the auditorium who may be some distance away at a large meeting. Use a consistent format with the title on each slide so that someone walking into the hall during your presentation will immediately be able to follow what you are saying. Make each statement short and relevant so that they will help the audience with their understanding of your paper and also give you a visual clue for what to say next. The use of colour will enhance the presentation but try to select the ones that project well. Everyone has a personal preference, but popular combinations are blue and white, and green and yellow. Dark backgrounds are less likely to show up blemishes on the slides. Always avoid using red text, as this is difficult to read.

Table 21.1   Rules for making good text slides

- Apply a simple consistent format and colour scheme:
  - Have the same heading on each slide;
  - Do not use more than five colours (except for histograms or graphs).
- Use a large type size.
- Avoid wide gaps between the lines of text.
- Use short punchy statements.
- Do not use more than eight words per line.
- Do not use more than six bulleted points.

Adapted from Lee (1995) with permission

Although transparencies may be cheaper and quicker to make than slides, they often give the impression of being done at the last minute. It is sometimes, but rarely, acceptable to use typewritten overheads, but never use those written by hand unless you actually want to draw on them at the time – in which case a computer presentation is preferable nowadays.

Data presented in a graph or chart is much easier to understand and remember than that given in a table. Follow the same rules as for the preparation of a text slide. Try not to include too much information and make the bars big enough to be seen from a distance. Graphs are extremely easy to prepare on the computer and will greatly enhance your presentation. It is usually simple to switch between the different formats of data presentation, such as a bar chart, pie chart or three-dimensional diagram. In general, two-dimensional bar charts are the simplest form for the audience to understand. Although 3D charts may sometimes look nice, they are often more difficult to comprehend and therefore your message may be missed. There is no excuse for using a table with a mass of data for which you have to 'apologise for this rather busy slide'. If there is an important point which you wish to make it is always worth reformatting the information (Thompson *et al.* 1987), putting the statistical significance in a different colour to draw attention to the significant results. A simple but essential aspect of data presentation is to make sure that your numbers all add up and correspond to those in your abstract. It is worthwhile remembering that there is usually someone who will be trying to catch you out.

The use of video, to show ultrasound images or a surgical procedure, frequently pleases the audience because it aids understanding and may give a research concept more clinical meaning. However, this will eat into the time available for your presentation, so it is always necessary to edit it down to the most important parts beforehand. Hospital medical photography departments are usually very helpful, if given plenty of notice, and it is always a good idea to be as friendly as possible towards them.

We find it difficult to recommend dual projection, especially for the inexperienced. Too often one of the carousels gets stuck or out of synchronisation, leading to much panic for the presenter and sometimes amusement for the audience. It is occasionally useful to show an ultrasound scan or picture with some text or a diagram, but never show two text slides at the same time.

Oral content
It is a mistake to spend too much time making the slides for a meeting and to forget about the oral content of the presentation (Table 21.2). The slides provide a backbone for your talk, but it is the way you present and discuss your arguments that is likely to win over an audience. To do this successfully, almost everyone needs to practice. Initially, you may wish to do this alone, perhaps in the lecture theatre at your own hospital or even in front of the mirror at home. It is then useful to ask a colleague or your boss to listen, so

Table 21.2   Essential steps in a good presentation

- Decide on your main message.
- Follow the rules for making slides.
- Mix text with pictures, tables and graphs.
- Practice until you feel confident.
- Maintain eye contact with the audience.
- Talk clearly in a friendly, relaxed but enthusiastic manner.
- Finish with a strong conclusion.

that they can identify any weak or confusing areas which need further work. They will also be able to help predict some potential questions, perhaps in areas which you had previously not considered. Use a clock or watch, so that you know how long the presentation is likely to take and can make the necessary adjustments. It is important not to overrun your allotted time as it looks unprofessional, reduces your discussion time and is not fair on the speaker who has to follow you. Good time-keeping is particularly important if you are the last person to present before coffee or lunch.

Sometimes you will be lucky enough to speak abroad at a meeting and there may be simultaneous translation. Remember than some English phrases are much longer when translated into a foreign language: '*John's hat*' is '*Il cappello di Giovanni*' in Italian. Other countries may not have an equivalent word for some medical terms or procedures (e.g. laparoscopy) and this means that the translator will have to provide a short description of the technique. As a basic principle, you can say far less if your talk is also being reproduced to a foreign audience, particularly if this is not being done on a professional basis. Translating your slides into the local language and presenting the same information in English can sometimes be a useful approach. It is always worth remembering that jokes can misfire when presenting overseas and they are, therefore, probably best avoided in this situation.

The first time you speak at an important meeting, you may feel more comfortable if you learn your talk 'by heart' in order to try to avoid drying up on 'the day.' This will give you much more confidence as the meeting approaches.

The meeting

It may seem obvious, but you must leave yourself plenty of time to travel to the meeting, especially if you are going to an unfamiliar city or using public transport. If you arrive on the day before, do not be tempted or persuaded by colleagues not giving a talk to stay out too late or drink alcohol, as you are unlikely to be at your best the following day.

Bear in mind the local climate or temperatures when selecting your clothing. Make sure you look good in a smart outfit with your hair combed.

Before your session starts, it is important to visit the lecture hall to get your bearings and look at how the console works. Check out how to change the slides and operate the lighting and pointer (Day 1995). If you are using glass-mounted slides, make sure they are kept at room temperature or they may be spoilt by distracting condensation marks. Double check that your slides are loaded the right way up and in the correct order. Well-organised conferences will have a preview room, which is enormously helpful. If possible, introduce yourself to the chairman.

The presentation

As the time for your talk approaches, it is likely that your pulse will quicken, palms become moist and mouth become dry. If this is usually a problem for you, ensure that a glass of water is available. When you are called to the podium walk confidently to the stage – this is your chance to impress. Attach the microphone to the lapel of your jacket and not your tie, as its movement often produces unnecessary background noise. Stand calmly, balanced on both feet, with your head up and your shoulders back. Use the title slide, not only to introduce the talk but also to give yourself time to settle. Say 'good morning' to your chairman and the audience, introduce yourself and the co-investigators or participants in your study. Perhaps follow this with a picture of your hospital or institution. Try to have a friendly, relaxed manner, as this will often help to get a favourable response. This is also necessary when things are not going as well as you would have hoped, for example when people walk in late or the pointer does not work. Always try to avoid appearing arrogant or over-confident, no matter how convinced you are that you are giving the perfect presentation, as this will alienate you from the audience, whom you should try to consider as your friends.

Your body language may be the cause of unnecessary distractions. To stop swaying or inappropriate arm movements, place one hand on the lectern. Do not flash the pointer around the hall. Eye contact is essential and you must look at the whole audience. Never turn sideways and start reading from the slides. Talk slowly and clearly, projecting your voice with plenty of energy so as to maintain the interest of the audience. If you look or sound bored, the audience may react in the same way. Vary the tone, pitch and volume of your presentation, perhaps with an occasional pause to emphasise a point. Sometimes it is worth asking a question, even if you answer it yourself. Try to avoid 'err err' and 'you know' – be fluent in what you have to say. Be aware of your dialect or accent and make sure you are understood.

Have something to add to each line of your text slides to ensure you do not just read them out. It is unnecessary to take a script or notes on to the podium. However, if you think you might forget essential figures, which you cannot fit on to the slides, take a card as an *aide memoire*. This is useful if there

Table 21.3 Points to be avoided in a presentation

Do not:

- Present too many ideas in too short a time.

- Use overheads or a new technique at an important meeting.

- Turn away from the audience and simply read your slides.

- Make distracting or inappropriate movements.

- Be over-confident, pompous or arrogant.

- Use too many slides too rapidly.

- Answer questions in a dismissive or confrontational manner.

- Run over your allotted time.

is a possibility that you will be asked technical or statistical questions in the discussion. As a general rule, you should use approximately one text slide for each minute (Lashford 1995) but you may use additional picture slides or illustrations. If your audience is unfamiliar with the topic or research methodology, use some link slides to make the lecture more understandable. Carefully talk people through the results, even if they are shown graphically. Explain the axes to the charts, the scales, what each bar shows and then, finally, the outcome of your study.

Try to maintain momentum throughout the talk and have a strong finish that summarises the main points. The conclusions are important because they contain the 'take home message' which is often the main thing people will remember. When you have finished, let the audience know by thanking them for their attention. Do not worry if you see a mass of hands raised to ask questions. This usually means you have generated some interest and is much better than having a silence, which may indicate that the audience were either bored or did not understand your presentation. Table 21.3 lists some of the points to be avoided in a presentation.

Answering the questions

If there are no questions, a good chairman will usually ask you something to get the ball rolling. Sometimes, someone in the audience will have found a particular aspect of your talk interesting and wish to have further information. Try to keep the audience on your side at this stage, even if you find the questioning aggressive or unfair. Thank the questioner for his comments, if appropriate, and then set about answering the question as you see fit. You will probably have anticipated some of the points during your preparation. If not, you should try and answer concisely while thinking on your feet. Do not make long, rambling statements which you have not thought through clearly.

Again, try to concentrate on the subject of your presentation and area of knowledge. It is usually unnecessary to make supplementary slides which can be used to answer anticipated questions, but it may be worthwhile if you feel there is a point worthy of expanding in the subsequent discussion.

If you are unsure of the answer to a question, say so and perhaps highlight areas where further work needs to be done. Sometimes the questioning is particularly tough and you may feel that your supervisor should be involved. Although this may seem an easy option, it often results in the debate going on around you with thoughts of your presentation sidelined. Try to answer the questions as best you can without bluffing and only ask for help as a last resort. The chairman will usually recognise that you are having some difficulties in a particular area and move the discussion on. It is vital that your presentation ends on a high note and a debate taking place in which you no longer have a part is a bad way to finish.

Conclusions

Presenting a paper at a meeting should be an exciting and stimulating experience, often at the end of months of scientific endeavour. Although you will quickly develop your own style of presentation, it is important to follow some basic rules so that your talk is a success. Start to prepare well in advance of the deadline. Define the main messages you wish to convey, make the appropriate slides and practice until you feel comfortable. On the day of the meeting, talk slowly and clearly in a confident but relaxed manner. Do not be over ambitious and never be pompous or arrogant. Use the slides to provide yourself with some visual reminders and the audience a framework for your study. Answer the questions succinctly, keeping a clear head and avoid confrontation where possible. Finally, try and look as though you are enjoying yourself no matter how terrified you feel inside!

References

Day, R.A. (1995) 'How to present a paper orally' in: R.A. Day (Ed.) *How to Write and Publish a Scientific Paper*, pp.144–147. Cambridge: Cambridge University Press

Lashford, L.S. (1995) Presenting a scientific paper, including the pitfalls. *Arch Dis Child* **73**, 168–9

Lee, N. (1995) Illustrating and presenting your data. ABC of Medical Computing. *BMJ* **311**, 319–22

Thompson, W.A., Mitchell, R.L., Halvorsen, R.A., Foster, W.L. and Roberts L. (1987) Scientific presentations. What to do and what not to do. *Invest Radiol* **22**, 224–45

## 22

How to set about writing your first paper

Philip N. Baker

Why bother?

Before starting your article, you need to identify what is motivating you to write your paper. You may have finished a study and feel that the findings are so important that they must be disseminated to as wide an audience as possible. Alternatively, you may feel that writing a paper will enhance both your CV and your future career prospects. Perhaps you need to silence your boss who is constantly nagging you to 'write up' a clinical finding. There are even some rare individuals who write papers because they enjoy writing! For many of you, there will be a combination of different factors motivating you to write this first paper – just reflect before you do so; does the paper merit your effort and will you be proud of the finished article?

Choice of journal

Before you start writing, it is a good idea to decide to which journal you are going to send your manuscript. The different journals require manuscripts written in particular styles and the choice of journal will govern the focus of the article. If the example of a study of a novel imaging technique in pregnancy were considered: a scientific journal would be most likely to accept a paper concerning the novelty of the technique, an article focused on the application of the technique to pregnancy should be sent to an obstetric clinical journal and a paper detailing the wider clinical applications might get into a general clinical journal. Unless you have a specific publication in mind, you should spend a few minutes browsing through the copies of journals kept at your local medical library.

The factors motivating you to write your paper will contribute to your choice of journal. In general, it is easier to get a paper published in a journal of low readership than in one which is widely read. Each journal has an 'impact factor' which indicates impact of papers published in the journal; that of the *Lancet* is higher than that of the *Archives of Gynaecology and Obstetrics*. You should be sensible – very few people have their first papers published in *Nature* or the *New England Journal of Medicine*, but there is little to be lost by aiming high. If your paper is rejected, you can always resubmit to a lesser journal.

After you have made your choice, you should obtain the instructions for authors which pertain to that journal. Journals vary; some publish these instructions in every issue, others on a yearly or six-monthly basis.

Title

When you read some of the titles of published articles, you get the impression that the authors have selected as esoteric a title as possible, in the hope that this will dissuade anyone from reading the paper. Other titles impart minimal information about the studies they describe. You are not writing a detective novel; the best titles start the paper by detailing the major result or finding of the work performed. There are, however, ways of emphasising the fact that your work is an original contribution. In an article on how to write 'nifty' titles, Yankelowitz (1980) suggested the following strategies:

- certain phrases imply soundness, such as 'A randomised trial of ... 'and 'Multiple linear regression analysis of...'
- some phrases suggest honesty, such as 'The failure of ... to influence ... ' and 'The unreliability of ... in assessing ...'
- others phrases sound innovative, such as 'The pathophysiological relationship between ... and ... : a hypothesis'; and 'The ... factor: a critical new parameter in examining ...'
- further phrases indicate a timely study, such as 'The relationship of ... to urban health care'.

Sadly, some papers never make it beyond the title stage, so press on.

Authorship

Your next decision concerns the authorship of the paper. The question of authorship of papers can occasionally be a source of conflict and potential authorship is best addressed before any writing commences and, indeed, before the research begins. If you have performed most of the work of the study and are writing the paper, then you will generally be the first author. The senior investigator, who is supervising both you and your study, will usually be the final author. Other individuals who have contributed to the study design, the work detailed in the study and the writing of the manuscript, may be entitled to be authors of your paper. The order of these authors should reflect their contribution to the study. Many papers list multiple authors and Quick (1969) discussed the problems of having eight or more authors in his poem entitled 'Number one *et al.*':

> It's two times four,
> And four times two,
> And what is more,
> Just who is who,
> Assuming one is the driving force,
> And number eight the chief, of course,

Then who is five,
What did he do,
That makes him five,
Instead of two,
Pity poor seven and six and three,
Their place suggests obscurity,
In time's recall,
Said paper shall,
Be known to all,
As such and such by one *et al.*

It is your job to ensure that all co-authors have made a valid contribution; many of the journals stipulate specific criteria for authorship. If you feel that an individual's efforts do not merit authorship, one alternative is to list their assistance in an acknowledgements section. For example, if a colleague simply allows access to patients, this would not merit authorship. It is also your responsibility to confirm that all co-authors have seen and approved a final version of the manuscript before it is submitted. Usually they will need to sign the letter accompanying submission or a copyright assignation.

Introduction

The introduction to the paper should explain why it was important that you performed the study. You should provide a brief background to the subject, focusing on the aspects under investigation. Although statements made in your introduction should be fully referenced, your readers should be able to comprehend your introduction without looking up the references. You should try to tailor the style of your introduction to the journal to which you are submitting. For example, if you are writing a paper on screening for Down syndrome, you will need to consider the importance of the details of prenatal diagnosis in greater depth if your paper is to be submitted to *Prenatal Diagnosis* than if you are planning to send it to the *British Medical Journal.*

Above all, your introduction should clearly state the question(s) you sought to answer and the hypothesis behind the study.

Methodology

The methodology section is often one of the easiest parts of the paper to write. It should contain a description of how you performed the study, with sufficient detail to enable any reader to repeat the study. If a particular aspect of the methodology has been described at length in a previous publication, it is appropriate to cite the previous manuscript and provide brief details. You should describe the measures that you have taken to validate the reliability of your techniques or assays. The exclusion and inclusion criteria of any patients studied should be described. Your methodology section may benefit from subheadings such as 'Specific methods', 'Patients studied' and 'Study design'.

You may need to pay particular attention to the statistical methods described in the paper. If you have any qualms regarding the validity of the statistics used in the study, you should discuss these with your co-authors or a statistician affiliated to your department.

Results

The findings of your study should be included in your results section. These findings may be in the form of tables, graphs or written text, and you should spend some time deciding which is the best way of presenting your data. It may be helpful to discuss the layout of your findings with either an experienced colleague or with somebody from your local audio visual department. You should try not to duplicate the presentation of your data in more than one form. The results of any statistical tests used to analyse your data should be included. The results section is not the place for any speculation or interpretation of your findings; leave any such considerations for the discussion.

Discussion

Your discussion section should consider whether the study has answered the questions which it was designed to address and whether the hypothesis proposed in the introduction has been proven or not. You should consider the implications of your study; for example, whether changes in clinical practice are supported or whether further studies are indicated. This section gives you the opportunity to speculate, to extrapolate from your findings and to discuss your results in relation to the previous literature, highlighting areas of agreement and attempting to explain areas of disagreement. You may wish to identify caveats to the study, or modifications which, in retrospect, would improve any future studies.

References

The references section is an important part of your paper and you will need to spend time and effort to ensure that this section is free from errors and omissions. An author that you have forgotten to quote, or have misinterpreted, may be the reviewer of your paper! Readers of your paper will rapidly become frustrated if they cannot find the references you have cited due to a typographical mistake. Different journals have different preferences regarding the style of reference citations and you should check that you comply with these before submitting your manuscript. The use of a reference manager software package will facilitate changing the style of your references should the paper be rejected and require a difference reference style (see Chapter 3).

Acknowledgements

This section allows you to acknowledge sponsors and collaborators who are not authors on the paper. It is particularly important for technicians with a major practical involvement in the paper or statisticians who have given time and effort to help you. Once the paper is published you should give them a copy of the paper with their acknowledgement detailed, as a useful way of retaining their co-operation in the future.

Abstract

Although the abstract precedes the introduction, you are probably best advised to defer writing the abstract until the rest of the paper is written. The abstract is arguably the most important part of the paper as more people will read it than will read the body of the paper. Your abstract should thus be as clear and as informative as possible. The abstract also needs to be concise and many journals impose a word limit. Some journals require abstracts to be in the form of a single paragraph. Others request structured abstracts which include the hypothesis or rationale of the study, specific methods/study design/setting, results (including the results of statistical tests) and a conclusion (the 'take-home' message of your study). Your best plan is to read a few abstracts in a recent copy of the journal to which you are submitting your manuscript, in order to get a good idea of what is needed.

Covering letter

Once the final draft of your paper is finished and all authors are satisfied, you should send the requisite number of copies to the editor of the journal. You should include a letter to the editor detailing your submission and explaining why the journal should consider your manuscript. The letter should include the statement that the work has not been published elsewhere and is not currently under consideration by another journal. If part of the work has been published in a meeting abstract, some journals require that a copy of that abstract should be submitted with the manuscript. The author identified for correspondence does not need to be the first author; if you are about to move hospitals it will be more sensible to choose one of your co-authors to correspond with the editor.

Journals vary markedly in their response times. At least two reviewers will assess your paper and you can only wait for the editor's reply.

The response

Responses from journals can be divided into three categories:
- an acceptance without modification
- an invitation to respond to the editor's or the reviewers' criticisms
- a rejection.

An acceptance without modification

It is unusual to have your first paper accepted without any changes being deemed necessary by the editor or reviewer. However, if you do receive such a positive response to your paper, bask in your success but do not assume that getting your papers accepted will always be so straightforward.

An invitation to respond to the editor's or the reviewers' criticisms

An invitation to respond to comments usually means that your paper will be accepted if you can address the points identified by the editor/reviewers to the editor's satisfaction. Unless the letter from the editor states that a revision will not be considered, a detailed response is likely to be successful. You need to examine each of the editor's/referees' comments in turn. Some of the criticisms are likely to be valid and sensible points, others may not be so reasonable. In your reply to the editor you should detail whether you have accepted each of the referees' comments (making the appropriate revision to your manuscript), or why the suggested alterations are inappropriate or unnecessary. It never does any harm to compliment the reviewer when the suggested amendments enhance your paper. The editor may then accept your paper or suggest further changes.

A rejection

While it is disappointing to have your paper rejected, you should not feel too downhearted. Just as many of the best novels, football players and recording artists were initially unappreciated, many papers are accepted by journals of higher quality than the original journal chosen. Again, you need to consider each of the criticisms made by the editor and reviewers. You should revise your manuscript in the light of comments which you feel are helpful and constructive. After discussion with your co-authors, you need to choose a journal to which to resubmit your paper. The paper may have been rejected because it was too clinical or too scientific for the journal originally chosen. Your manuscript will probably need to be revised in order to comply with the journal's specifications. If your paper is repeatedly rejected, you do need to reflect whether publication is merited.

Proofs

Shortly before your accepted paper is published, the corresponding author will receive proof copies from the printer. Despite months having passed from your original submission, you will be expected to respond in 48–72 hours. You should read the proof copies and carefully amend any typographical errors. No major changes can be made to the paper at this stage. The proof copies need to be returned to the publisher, even when no alterations are necessary. Failure to return proof copies has delayed the publication of papers by months.

References
Yankelowitz, B.Y. (1980) How to write nifty titles for your papers. *BMJ* **1**, 96
Quick, D.J. (1969) Number one *et al. New Engl J Med* **281**, 911

## 23

How a paper is reviewed and why it might be turned down

John M. Grant
and Allison Laird

Virtually all medical and scientific journals accept papers for publication only after rigorous peer review, for there is evidence that peer review improves the scientific quality of the papers published by a journal. Journals vary in their policies regarding peer review. Weekly medical journals with large circulations have a permanent staff of scientific editors who will often reject a paper without external peer review and only send to referees those papers which overcome this initial hurdle (for example, the *British Medical Journal*). Most medical journals, however, including the *British Journal of Obstetrics and Gynaecology* (BJOG), belong to societies, are published monthly and do not have a permanent staff of scientific editors. Society journals, therefore, send virtually every manuscript for external peer review. Some authors find it comforting that their paper will be assessed by an expert; others disconcerting, for there are concerns about bias in the judgement of papers, sometimes conflicts of intellectual interest and sometimes what are called 'conflicts of passion'. The wise editor will choose referees who are analytical and constructive and who are unlikely to show bias, even if this means finding a referee outside the UK. Some journals insist that, as far as possible, the authors and the referees should be unaware of each other's identity. Other journals reveal the identity of authors and referees to each other. The *BJOG* take a middle course, masking the identity of the authors to the referees, but encouraging the referees to sign their reports. This practice may seem illogical, but it is based on the results of a randomised trial by McNutt *et al.* (1990), who found that concealing the identity of the authors resulted in a higher standard of referees' reports, while authors preferred the referees' reports to be signed, finding them more constructive and more courteous.

The editorial process

Figure 23.1 shows the editorial process at the *BJOG*. Each manuscript is sent to two clinical referees. If both referees agree that the paper is scientifically flawed we send a polite rejection letter. If even one referee suggests that the paper has some scientific merit we send the paper to one of five editors for discussion at the next monthly meeting. About half the papers discussed at the meeting which are turned down are rejected because, although there may be nothing intrinsically wrong with them, they are thought to be too

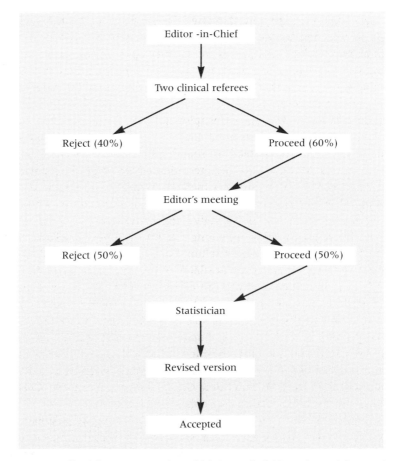

Figure 23.1 Editorial processes at the *British Journal of Obstetrics and Gynaecology*

technical, too specialised or to have too little interest for our readers. If papers pass this hurdle, they may be sent to a statistician if they contain numerical comparisons, following which the clinical and statistical reports are sent to the authors with recommendations on improving the paper. When the revised version is received, provided the referees' and editors' questions have been answered satisfactorily, a formal acceptance letter is sent.

Many authors complain about what they perceive as the apparent slowness of the editorial procedures. However, authors themselves often contribute to delay in two important ways: by failing to adhere to the 'instructions to authors', which are found in every issue, and by failing to present their work in clear, precise, unambiguous, grammatically correct English, which is free from jargon and an alphabet soup of acronyms. Most delays of this sort are due to sloppiness, both in attention to detail (i.e. submission requirements or to the references) and in expression of thought. The former is amenable to correction, but the latter can be fatal, for clarity in writing is a direct reflection of clarity in thinking. Good scientific research is often doomed to rejection by the chaos of language in which it is lost. Authors sometimes object when their papers are returned again and again for revision, claiming bias. And they are right: we have a very strong bias *in favour of* publishing good science that is well written. We will not publish papers inadequately revised or poorly presented.

Although large weekly journals employ full-time technical editors for the task of rendering papers into good English, the result is an amorphous product in which all papers tend to 'sound alike'. This, we feel, is similarly unfair to authors. Moreover, as these technical editors tend to be individuals with medical degrees, they are an expensive luxury which society journals cannot afford. At the *BJOG* every effort is made to assist authors whose first language is not English. But increasingly – and alarmingly – we find that those most culpable of poor writing are young registrars or research fellows whose first language is English – those for whom essays are no longer requirements. However, we believe it is the responsibility of the authors to write the paper so clearly as to be understood without difficulty and those who feel it is the job of the editors to re-write the paper for them are gravely mistaken.

We recommend that authors consult *Hart's Rules for Compositors* (Oxford University Press) and *The Uniform Requirements for Manuscripts Submitted to Medical Journals* (International Committee of Medical Journal Editors). There are also a number of useful guides to scientific writing available at university bookshops or from the BMJ Publishing Group, which may provide assistance in writing effectively for medical journals.

The process is time consuming, but we feel that these procedures are necessary in order to safeguard our standards of scientific integrity. On average it takes about five months for a paper to be accepted for the BJOG. Altogether, it will take, on average, nine months to appear in print after receipt. We make no apology for this time, for we prefer to publish good science slowly than poor science quickly. Besides, the time taken to publish a paper is typical of all monthly journals, for compared with weekly journals they have only a quarter of the opportunities to publish.

Publishing criteria

You will have realised from these paragraphs that the aim of the *BJOG* is to publish the highest quality scientific research in obstetrics and gynaecology and women's health. We do publish review articles to educate, commentaries to provoke and correspondence to answer provocation, but together these constitute less than one-tenth of the pages we publish. Our aim is to publish original research which is important to women's health. We have three main criteria by which we accept papers for publications:

- originality
- scientific merit
- clinical importance.

The most important of these is scientific merit. These criteria are, therefore, not given equal weight: a basic science article should be original and scientifically sound, but its clinical importance may not be obvious; while a randomised trial should be clinically important and scientifically sound, but need not be original, for its results may be included in a systematic review.

Basic science

We publish both basic science and clinical research, of which basic science is the more important, for it is only through basic science that we can increase our understanding of the pathophysiology of disease and its treatment. Yet, paradoxically, most of the articles on basic science we receive are scientifically poor and badly presented. We shall illustrate this with an imaginary study (for we do not wish to offend anyone by describing a paper we have actually rejected).

Pre-eclampsia is a condition in which damage occurs to endothelium. Endothelin is a polypeptide within endothelium which constricts smooth muscle in small arteries. Endothelial damage in pre-eclampsia releases endothelin, which may, therefore, be the cause of the vasoconstriction and hypertension in this condition. Is the concentration of endothelin in the plasma increased in pre-eclampsia? To test this hypothesis the investigators took samples of blood from 20 women with pre-eclampsia and 20 women without pre-eclampsia who acted as controls. The results of this imaginary study are shown in Table 23.1, where the endothelin concentrations are compared by a t-test, from which the authors conclude that the concentration of endothelin is not increased in pre-eclampsia. Is this conclusion justified? It is not, for there are many problems with the design and analysis of this study and the presentation of its results.

- In Table 23.1, *n* in the group with pre-eclampsia is 44 when it should be 20. It is obvious that the investigators, so enthusiastic were they that endothelin really was responsible for the vasoconstriction of pre-eclampsia, took several samples from the women with pre-eclampsia throughout pregnancy and included the results from all the samples in

Table 23.1	Pitfalls in the presentation of results	
	Pre-eclampsia	**Controls**
n	44	20
Age	21.6 ± 1.6	26.5 ± 1.3
Parity	0.3 ± 0.6	1.3 ± 0.6
Gestational age	34.2 ± 1.2	38.1 ± 1.2
Endothelin	1.6 ± 1.5	0.8 ± 0.9[a]
[a] *P* = NS		

the analysis. This is a mistake, for the results from several samples taken from the same woman are not independent of one another and will therefore introduce a bias into the study. The unit of analysis is the woman, not the sample. The investigators should have selected one sample only from each woman – the last sample, one chosen at random, or the mean of all the samples for each woman.

- In Table 23.1, no units of measurement are given for any of the variables. We can deduce that age is in years and gestational age in weeks, but what is the unit of measurement of endothelin?
- Parity is not a continuous variable and the correct method of presentation is 'nulliparae n (%); multiparae n (%)'.
- Inspection of Table 23.1 shows that the women with pre-eclampsia were younger, their pregnancies were earlier and that there were more nulliparae than the controls. It is possible that endothelin concentrations in the plasma depend on maternal age, gestational age and parity, such that the investigators should have chosen the control group with much more care, to match these possible confounding variables.
- The information in Table 23.1 suggests measurements of central tendency and dispersion of the data, but we do not know whether central tendency is expressed as the mean, median or mode, and the '±' notation is not explained, whether standard error or standard deviation. In their instructions to authors, virtually all scientific journals do not accept the '±' notation because of this confusion. The preferred description is to add a note to Table 23.1: 'Numbers are mean (SD) (let us assume they are mean and standard deviation), or n (%)'.
- The investigators have performed a t-test to compare the endothelin concentrations in each group, but it is obvious that the standard deviations are very large compared with the means, suggesting that the data do not follow a normal distribution. A t-test is therefore inappropriate, the correct procedure being a Mann–Whitney U-test. In presenting the results of the Mann–Whitney test it is insufficient to say 'P = NS'; the Mann–Whitney U-statistic should be stated, with the actual P value. Notwithstanding the results of the statistical test it is more informative for readers if the endothelin concentrations are presented graphically, either as a dot plot or a box-and-whisker plot. Graphical presentation allows the reader to appreciate visually the distribution of the data and to perceive any difference between the groups.
- Inspection of the mean endothelin concentrations in Table 23.1 shows that there really may be a difference in endothelin concentrations, but that the study was too small to show that this difference is statistically significant. The investigators should have estimated the size of study required to be able to show a difference between the two groups which was statistically significant.

We have no knowledge concerning the functions of endothelin and we do not even know in what units it is measured and it may be that the hypothesis tested in this imaginary study is biologically implausible. Nevertheless, we would have no hesitation in rejecting this paper without sending it to a referee, because of the fatal flaws in the design and analysis of the study it describes, and the letter of rejection would include these seven points. If, however, the study was well designed and analysed we would then send the paper to a referee with knowledge of the subject, to assess its originality and if possible its clinical importance.

The majority of the papers we receive are concerned with clinical research but, again, problems with their design and analysis are common. Audit is a favourite topic, for we are obliged by our hospital trusts to be involved with audit, yet the *BJOG* rarely publishes papers on audit, for scientific reasons.

Audit

Figure 23.2 illustrates an imaginary audit. A maternity unit is concerned at its high rate of caesarean sections – 16% – and a survey is undertaken to establish the reasons for performing caesarean section. The main reason is slow labour, so guidelines are formulated for the treatment of this complication. After a year another survey is performed, when the caesarean section rate is found to be 12%. The chief executive of the trust is effusive in his congratulations and everyone enjoys a night out to celebrate this achievement, when someone mentions that it would be a good idea to send a paper to the *BJOG*, as he is sure they will be interested in the results of the audit.

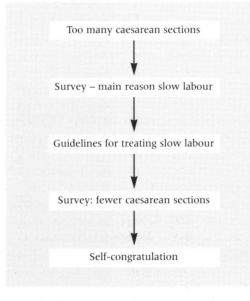

Figure 23.2 Audit of caesarean section

Table 23.2 The fallacy of audit		
	1997	**1998**
Caesarean section rate	16%	12%
Parity		
primiparae	40%	30%
nulliparae	60%	70%
Induction of labour	25%	15%
CTG tutorials	No	Yes
Perinatologist	Yes	No

It would not be published. The reasons can be determined from Table 23.2, which shows the spectacular reduction in the rate caesarean sections. However, between the two surveys a peripheral maternity hospital caring for women at low risk of complications closed, with the transfer of these women to the main maternity unit. This transfer resulted in an increase in the proportion of multiparae delivered in the maternity unit, who have a lower chance of caesarean section. Also in that year there was a decline in the number of women undergoing induction of labour consequent upon a disaster with vaginal prostaglandin; induction of labour is associated with an increased risk of caesarean section. There was also a difficult legal case concerning birth asphyxia, which resulted in regular formal tutorials in the interpretation of fetal heart-rate traces. The number of caesarean sections for supposed fetal distress declined, perhaps because of increased familiarity with the pathophysiology of fetal hypoxia. In the previous year, the unit boasted a perinatologist who later sought advancement elsewhere. This is associated with less risk of caesarean section, for it is known that tertiary referral centres have higher rates of caesarean section than district hospitals, when similar cases are compared.

There is, therefore, little justification for supposing that the reduction in caesarean section rate in 1998 is due to the newly formulated guidelines for treating slow labour, as it could be due to other changes in clinical practice and changes in the type of pregnant woman cared for by the maternity unit. The problem with audit is that it relies on historical controls and is therefore subject to bias. The biases in this imaginary audit are obvious. However, often they are so subtle as to be barely perceptible, but they may have a significant effect on an outcome. The aim of the BJOG is the publication of the highest quality scientific research in obstetrics and gynaecology; we therefore cannot publish audit, because of its biases. Audit is not science. Audit may be useful to suggest hypotheses which may then be tested. For example, it may be possible to perform a trial of the guidelines for treating slow labour where maternity units are randomised to receive the guidelines or not and then measure the difference in caesarean section rate. Audit may then become science.

The lesson for young researchers is that you will not improve your curriculum vitae by local audit projects, for when you apply for an academic post in a teaching hospital audit will not count. You should not waste your earthly substance on audit. Audit is important to the managers of hospital trusts and we all have to be involved in audit, but audit should be kept separate from scientific research.

Surveys of clinical practice

Another favourite topic of clinical research is questionnaire surveys of clinical practice, for these appear to be easy to perform. It is possible, on payment of a small fee, to obtain a list of the names and addresses of all obstetricians and gynaecologists in the UK and then to send a questionnaire asking about their clinical practice. We rarely publish questionnaire surveys of this sort.

Table 23.3 shows the results of the first question of an imaginary survey sent to all 1300 consultant gynaecologists in the UK, asking about their treatment of excessive menstruation. From this survey the investigators concluded that consultant gynaecologists were not practising evidence-based medicine derived from meta-analyses of randomised trials, as they were not prescribing tranexamic acid often enough, were prescribing norethisterone too often, were not using the levonorgestrel–intrauterine system enough, were not performing endometrial ablation enough and were performing far too many hysterectomies. A shocking state of affairs. The authors conclude that we need national guidelines for the treatment of excessive menstruation. This would be followed by headlines in the tabloid press *'Gynaecologists too knife-happy. Minister to make a statement'*.

This paper would not be published. Table 23.4 shows that not only did half the gynaecologists not respond to the survey, but that the responders were different from the non-responders. The responders were older, more years

---

Table 23.3 Bias in surveys of medical practice

A woman aged 40 attends your clinic with excessive menstruation. What is the first treatment you would offer?

Tranexamic acid	35	(5%)
Norethisterone	215	(30%)
Levonorgestrel intrauterine system	72	(10%)
Endometrial ablation	107	(15%)
Hysterectomy	286	(40%)

Table 23.4 Faults with this survey: responders versus non-responders

	Responders (%)		Non-responders (%)	
n	715	(55)	585	(45)
Age (years)	54.1	(5.6)	43.9	(7.6)
Years since MRCOG	23.3	(5.4)	14.8	(7.6)
Hospital:				
teaching	429	(60)	234	(40)
district	286	(40)	351	(60)
Subspeciality interest in				
gynaecology	238	(33)	390	(67)
Numbers are mean (SD) or n (%).				

had elapsed since they passed the MRCOG, a greater proportion worked in teaching hospitals and a lesser proportion had a subspeciality interest in gynaecology. It is likely that the non-responders, had they responded, would have answered the questions differently. Table 23.5 shows even greater sources of bias, for when a single set of case notes for each responder was randomly selected, actual practice was found to be quite different from the stated practice. This is not surprising, for a consultant gynaecologist does not treat women in isolation, but he is assisted in his clinic by registrars and staff-grade gynaecologists who may have different practices concerning the treatment of excessive menstruation. In this imaginary survey, Table 23.5 shows that actual clinical practice follows the results of randomised trials much more closely than the stated practice. The Minister can rest in peace.

It is possible to undertake surveys of clinical practice which are scientifically sound. Instead of performing a survey of all consultant gynaecologists in the UK, a random sample should be chosen, stratified for age and type of hospital, teaching or district. Non-responders should be followed up by two reminder letters. The characteristics of the responders and the non-responders

Table 23.5 Faults with this survey: responders – stated versus actual practice

Treatment	Stated	(%)	Actual	(%)
Tranexamic acid	35	(5)	70	(10)
Norethisterone	215	(30)	108	(15)
Levonorgestrel intrauterine system	72	(10)	144	(20)
Endometrial ablation	107	(15)	214	(30)
Hysterectomy	286	(40)	179	(25)

should be compared, to identify biases. A survey of a random sample of case notes should be carried out, to ascertain how far actual practice agrees with the stated practice. A survey of clinical practice is very time consuming and costly and cannot be undertaken lightly. We receive many surveys of clinical practice, but few are published.

Elimination of bias

By now you will have realised that the theme of this chapter is bias and the elimination of bias, both in the design of a scientific project and in the peer review of a paper. The elimination of bias is the key to publication in a scientific journal. The simplest types of study are more likely to be published in a journal, because they are free of bias. We publish case reports, provided they are original and are clinically important. It is often thought that, with case series, the chances of publication are increased if there is a control group. The opposite is true, as the selection of suitable controls is difficult and the introduction of a control group in order to make numerical comparisons invites bias. An uncontrolled case series has much more chance of publication as, without a comparison with a control group, there is no risk of bias. We sometimes receive a paper describing a case series with concurrent or historical controls when, if the case series is interesting, we may ask for the control group to be removed. Uncontrolled case series are useful for describing a new technique or a new complication of a new or an established technique and suggest hypotheses which can be tested in a randomised trial. Recently, we have published uncontrolled case series of endometrial ablation and the levonorgestrel–intrauterine system for the treatment of excessive menstruation, suggesting the next step of a randomised trial to compare the two methods. The strongest scientific evidence comes from randomised trials, as the process of randomisation eliminates the biases between the groups of women being compared. You will have the greatest chance of publication if you participate in a randomised trial – provided it is well designed.

References

McNutt, R.A., Evans, A.T., Fletcher, R.H. and Fletcher, S.W. (1990) The effects of blinding on the quality of peer review. A randomized trial. *JAMA* **263**, 1371–6

Further reading

Hart's Rules (1983) *Hart's Rules for Compositors and Readers*. Oxford: Oxford University Press

The Uniform Requirements for Manuscripts Submitted to Medical Journals, available free of charge from the Secretariat Office of the International Committee of Medical Journal Editors in Philadelphia, Pennsylvania, USA. Tel. 800–523–1546 ext. 2660.

## 24

How to prepare a thesis

J. Jonathan O. Herod

Introduction

It is said that people learn by their mistakes, but a wise man learns by the mistakes of others. So, if you are contemplating doing some research and writing a thesis, here is a chance to get wise before the event. Everyone is familiar with the person who is 'busy writing up my MD' often many years after finishing their research. Sadly, the majority of these people will never complete this task but will waste huge amounts of their time in failing to do so. Furthermore, the unfinished thesis will become a considerable millstone around their neck instead of a great advantage and achievement. The important question is – how can this state of affairs be avoided?

Having made every mistake in the book, I hope this chapter may assist others in avoiding them. Indeed, this is not such a difficult task but simply involves a bit of planning before starting and sticking to objectives and goals with determination. This chapter is very much my personal view. The next chapter explains in detail the areas required by an examiner and it is essential that Chapter 25 is read in conjunction with this one.

Before you start

Most people commencing a period of time in research will be joining an established unit either to continue work already started or to begin a project which follows on from previous studies within that unit. They may be somewhat familiar with the background to the work but often they will be embarking on studies in a relatively unfamiliar area. Therefore, prior to commencing the actual work, either in a laboratory or in a clinical setting, it is vital to spend some time carrying out preparatory work. Time spent in this preparatory phase will be rewarded many times over at a later date.

The first objective is to meet with one's supervisor to discuss the proposed project in detail. Supervisors, like any group of people, vary enormously and the particular characteristics and abilities of the supervisor will have a great impact on the ease or difficulty with which the work is completed. While one may be fortunate and have the world's greatest supervisor, this will obviously not be the rule. Therefore, prior to any discussion, time should be spent considering exactly what information is required. The sensible person will write down the relevant questions and attend this meeting with what amounts to an agenda for discussion. See Chapter 18 for a detailed discussion of supervising and being supervised.

It is important to find out about the background to, and the aims of the current investigation in as much detail as possible. If anything is not clear, as is usual at this stage, then one should not be afraid to say so. It is particularly useful to try to establish a proposed time frame for the study, with goals that should be met at specified intervals within the overall period of research. This is also the time to find out exactly what is required of the researcher in terms of the thesis that will be produced. It may be helpful to obtain a copy of a recently completed thesis as a guide, or to seek the advice of someone who has recently completed their thesis. Many universities now have formal guidelines for the format of theses and these should be consulted early on. One should also determine who else, in addition to the supervisor, will be involved in the work and it would be worthwhile to meet and discuss the project with all of these individuals at the earliest opportunity.

Having completed this preliminary step it is time to retire, contemplate and then write down one's own plan of action and to set realistic achievement targets. This plan of action should be something which is referred to and adhered to throughout the time of the study.

It is tempting, at this stage, to throw oneself directly into the research project itself but again this would be a mistake. It is important that, prior to commencing the work, a detailed literature search should be completed and that time should be spent carefully reading and digesting the information collected. There are a number of reasons why it is advantageous to do this prior to commencing work on the project. First, it is often the case that research work becomes all-consuming. If preparatory work is not completed before commencing work, it may be neglected until it is too late. Secondly, in order to complete a project efficiently one must have a thorough under-standing of the area of investigation. It may be that information gathered at this stage will prevent many wasted hours by once again helping to avoid making mistakes that have previously been made by others. Lastly, it is a much quicker process to get the chore of finding all the relevant literature out of the way in one go, rather than attempting to do it piecemeal once there are other distractions competing for one's time.

It is likely that some important references will have been provided by one's supervisor, but there really is no substitute for spending time in the best library available (see Chapter 5). The process of searching the literature has been revolutionised in the last decade with the advent of widely available computerised facilities which assist in the process. The majority of postgrad-uate libraries will have a system which allows one to search for articles containing relevant keywords, authors and so on, at the touch of a button. These computer programs are simple to use but help from the library staff is usually readily available for the uninitiated. Often, the system will allow one to view an abstract from most articles and to save and print out all the titles relevant to the area of research. Then all that is required is to find the articles, photocopy them and go and read them straight away. If they are left on the floor in a pile in the corner it will become harder and harder to read them.

One word of advice regarding photocopying may be in order here. In the present economic climate it is likely that most researchers will have to fund the costs of reproducing articles from their own pocket. The more frugal individual may attempt to save money by using the reducing facility available on a photocopier or by printing articles on larger paper so that more pages can be fitted on to each sheet of paper used. However, the small amount of money saved is little recompense for the extra difficulties that occur when trying to read minuscule, poorly reproduced print or when manhandling large pieces of paper. It is likely that notes will need to be made all over these papers, so it is more efficient to use one sheet of A4 paper per page.

Once the articles have been read, it will become apparent that no literature search programme is ever complete. There will undoubtedly be a number of previously unidentified articles which are discovered and these articles should also be located, reproduced and read before commencing the project itself. In addition, relevant work will be published during the time that the research is carried out and, hence, it is worthwhile to take time every few months to search for any recently published work that is relevant. However, having completed this task, the eager reader will be pleased to learn that it is now time for the real work to begin.

Writing the thesis

Writing a thesis may at first sight seem a somewhat daunting task, no matter how skilled or rapid a writer one is. It is certain that this task does not seem any smaller with time and, indeed, the converse may well be true. Therefore, it is best to begin the writing process at the earliest possible opportunity with the aim that the bulk of the writing of the thesis, i.e. the introduction and methods sections, should be completed well before completion of the work itself. Starting early is a good way of harnessing the enthusiasm and optimism that most people experience at the start of a research project. It is also the optimal way of developing a thorough understanding of all aspects of the topic under investigation. Perhaps most importantly, it should be recognised that one's chances of completing the thesis at the end of the work will be greatly enhanced if the bulk of the writing has been completed at an early stage and one's quality of life will be immeasurably improved in the long run.

How to write

No one method will suit all people when it comes to writing any piece of work, but few find it an easy task. Everyone is familiar, to a greater or lesser extent, with writer's block. All of us have sat down at a desk and spent an hour or more agonising over the exact phrasing of an opening sentence or sometimes, sadly, of the title. This is a demoralising experience which leads to much wasted time and, all too often, the problem becomes repetitive in nature. There follows a description of my own approach which I hope will be helpful to readers.

This approach can be described in four phases:

- preparation
- writing
- fine tuning
- references.

Preparation

The preparatory phase is aimed at making writing easier by turning the writing from one large daunting task into a series of much smaller, less daunting, sequential tasks. It could be simply described as making a very detailed 'essay plan'. The first step is make a rough outline of the topics that will be covered in the thesis and to arrange them in an appropriate order. It would be worth discussing this outline with one's supervisor prior to commencing. Each of these topics can then be addressed in turn. Start by finding all the relevant articles for the first topic and numbering them. Next, take a red pen or fluorescent marker and carefully read through each article, marking all the interesting and relevant areas. During this reading phase, it is possible to build up a detailed plan of what will be said and to note alongside the plan which of the numbered articles give information about each particular part of the plan. The more detailed this plan becomes, the easier the task of writing will become. If a computer or word processor is to be used for writing (and this is essential – see below) then the plan should be made on it.

Writing

As mentioned above, most people do not find writing easy, but it is something that simply has to be done. There is, however, one cardinal rule about writing which can be summed up as: always write something. What this means is that sitting staring over a blank piece of paper is one of the worst ways of wasting one's life away. When faced with the legendary 'writer's block' there are only two sensible options: either go away and do something more useful or write something down. The problem probably arises because of a desire to write everything perfectly at the first attempt. However, it is a certainty that the first draft written will always differ substantially from the final draft and it is much easier to edit and improve the odd badly written paragraph than to edit a blank piece of paper.

A great aid to the writing process is to use a computer with a word-processing package. It is so much easier to write when one knows that the text can be altered ad infinitum. It is strange how much better a piece of writing may appear on a computer screen, in hard type, than in one's own scruffy handwriting. My own preference is to start a piece of work with a heading at the top, a small space in which to write and my 'essay plan' at the bottom. As each part of the essay plan is accomplished, that line is cut and pasted on to the bottom of the plan, which helps to give the sensation that progress is being made.

Fine tuning

As stated above, the final version of a thesis is likely to differ substantially from an initial draft. Once a first draft is completed it should be spell-checked and then printed out and rechecked for the spelling and grammatical mistakes which are present, before being given to a third party (usually one's supervisor) for scrutiny and suggestions as to how the work can be improved. This process may involve more than one other person and may have to be repeated a number of times before the thesis is completed satisfactorily, although the fine-tuning process is much less laborious than the initial writing.

References

Referencing is an important part of any thesis. It is also an undoubtedly time-consuming and somewhat tedious task. One should first of all determine the format of referencing which will be required, as having to redo referencing in a different style is an unnecessary and soul-destroying task. Rather than leaving the references until the written work has been completed, it is more efficient to be diligent about recording them as an integral part of the writing process. Many individuals will have to complete this task by hand, but for those who use a computer for their writing, a number of referencing programs are now available. These will greatly reduce the workload and, wherever possible, it is worthwhile to make an effort to acquire the necessary software before beginning the task of writing. Whatever method is used, however, attention to detail is of primary importance. All examiners will check a proportion of the references cited and they dislike omissions as indicating a general sloppiness of approach.

Results and statistical analysis

As with all the processes of preparing a thesis, some thought given to the recording and analysis of results before commencing work will pay a great dividend at a later date. Huge amounts of results may be produced during the work carried out and often fairly sophisticated analysis will be required. Most researchers will not be gifted statisticians and statistical help from an expert will often be required. If this is the case, it is important to meet with the person who will give statistical assistance prior to commencing the work itself.

The information which is important will, of course, differ according to the nature of the work undertaken (see Chapters 14 and 16).

Whatever form of work is carried out, it is important to be diligent about recording data. As with writing, the longer the process is ignored, the harder it will become to begin the task. It would be sensible to set aside time each week to record any results produced during that week. This will once again reduce one large difficult task into a series of smaller, much easier tasks. Remember to be careful about the labelling of results and to record detailed accounts of the methods used in experimental work. Abbreviations and incomplete information which may seem perfectly explanatory at the time of writing are often baffling when reviewed at a later date.

Presentation of the results is one of the most important parts of the thesis. Again, take the advice of as many people as possible regarding how this task should be approached. A helpful statistician is invaluable in this respect and reference to other theses presenting similar types of data is obviously a great help. It should also be remembered that many departments now have access to excellent illustrative departments whose expertise may be invaluable.

Writing conclusions

Writing one's concluding thoughts should be the final task, if the bulk of the thesis has been completed early as suggested. This is clearly an area which should be discussed thoroughly with the person supervising the work before proceeding to writing. The majority of work carried out will not produce earth-shattering results, but negative results should be regarded with equal importance as positive ones. Beware of making claims which cannot be justified by the results produced and remember that it is important to write a balanced appraisal of the work which has been completed. It is of particular importance to address the shortcomings as well as the strengths of the work which has been performed and to consider how the work may be improved or where future work could continue the investigation.

Putting the thesis together

Once all the hard work has been completed, all that remains is to produce the thesis itself. This task is often surprisingly time-consuming, but it is important to do this carefully and to pay attention to detail. Remember to study carefully details of the format required by the assessing body. It is likely that stipulations will be made regarding the fonts used and spacing of lines and so on. These details may seem trivial but should not be overlooked. Again, reference to a completed thesis submitted recently is useful and will help with ideas about how the thesis should be structured. Once the thesis has been assembled it should again be presented to one's supervisor prior to binding, so that no errors should be overlooked.

Summary

Writing a thesis is a task which should not be underestimated, and is one which will almost always take considerably longer than expected. The wise person will, therefore, use the help of as many people as possible at all stages of the process. The value of preparatory work cannot be overstated and this work should ideally be completed before commencing the investigative work itself, as it will be hard to complete once the work is under way. As much of the writing as possible should be undertaken during the period of time that the work is being carried out, as leaving this process until the completion of that work leaves a daunting and dispiriting task to be tackled. These points may seem very simplistic, but adherence to them will maximise one's chances of completing a thesis and minimise the undoubted effort involved.

## 25

How a thesis or dissertation is assessed or examined

Fiona Broughton Pipkin

The examiners

By the time a thesis or dissertation is submitted, the candidate will have expended much time, effort and thought on it. The thesis is meant to display not only the results of a piece of original research but also a wide general knowledge of the field of study in which the subject matter lies. It will therefore be examined by two or more examiners or assessors, each of whom will be expert in all or a part of the subject matter. The examiners will almost always themselves have research degrees and are, therefore, in something of the position of a poacher turned gamekeeper. Having been there themselves, they can recognise evasions and omissions with considerable ease. There will always be one internal examiner who will usually come from the same department as that in which you have done your work, although he or she may sometimes come from another department in the faculty or indeed from another faculty within the university. There will also be at least one external examiner. This is an attempt to ensure that common standards for acceptance of work to a Masters or Doctoral level are imposed across the United Kingdom. Once suitable names have been identified and agreed by your supervisor and head of department, the potential examiners will be contacted informally to ascertain their willingness to act. This is not usually done until you are very close to submitting your thesis. These days, examiners are usually asked only to undertake the examination of a piece of work if they can complete it within a stated period, usually a maximum of three to four months. Practice varies between universities as to whether or not the candidate is given the name of his or her examiners before their thesis is submitted.

What follows is based on my own practice when examining theses. Individual examiners will have their own ways of doing things, but most will follow the broad outline detailed below. I have used the word 'thesis' throughout to describe a coherent piece of writing relating to a research project submitted in whole or in part in completion of the requirements for the award of a higher degree, usually at Doctoral level. Although a dissertation is a smaller work, the principles remain the same.

Examining the thesis

My first impressions of the thesis are important. Many universities today allow the submission of a ring-bound document, rather than expecting candidates to go to the expense of having the thesis hard bound at first attempt. This is because it is very unusual for a thesis to be allowed to go through with no requirement for amendments. With the near-universal use of word processors and photocopiers, there is no excuse for the submission of a dog-eared typescript with manuscript corrections. If you cannot be bothered with the physical appearance of your work, I may immediately begin to wonder how much you have bothered about its execution. I will have a preliminary look at the thesis, usually on the day on which I receive it. I will then allocate quality time to read it, setting aside one, or at the most two, clearly defined periods where I will concentrate on nothing else. You will have spent a long time working on your thesis; it is only reasonable that I should give it my undivided attention. When I settle down to the first reading, I do my best to ensure that my telephone does not ring and that I am not disturbed.

The title

The title should be succinct and informative. Ideally, I like to see an abstract of the thesis before deciding whether or not to agree to examine it. However, this is not often provided and my decision will therefore be based on the title and my knowledge of the department from which the work has come. If the title turns out to be misleading, then I am immediately slightly disposed against the thesis.

The introduction

The introduction should focus on the background to the study and not, for instance, be a general overview of obstetrics or gynaecology. I expect it to demonstrate wide background reading and a critical faculty on your part. I do not expect such comments as 'Smith *et al.* found 'x' but Brown *et al.* could not confirm this' without some attempt to explain why the two groups differed. I do not expect to read sentence after sentence telling me that more or less the same thing has been described by nine or ten research groups. Under these circumstances, I want to see one summary sentence with the appropriate referencing. I am looking for evidence of your capacity to synthesise or bring together data from many papers in a clear, accurate and intelligible manner and to view it critically. In any project with a bench-based component, you will need to demonstrate your familiarity not only with current techniques but also with those in use 10 or 15 years ago. Many apparent discrepancies in data can be accounted for in terms of changes in methodology. I look for 'signposts' to areas which you find interesting or unresolved questions which will point me in the direction of your thesis work. The introduction must make clear how and why the objectives of the work have been arrived at and therefore why the study is interesting.

Aims and objectives

I expect to see a clear and formal statement of aims and objectives. Practice varies between universities, but this is usually presented either as a separate section before the introduction or at the end of the introduction. You should be aware that, when I have finished reading the thesis, I am also looking for a summary of conclusions showing how you have attempted to attain each of the objectives outlined at this point.

Methods

The methods section must be given in sufficient detail to allow someone of comparable background to repeat the work. I look for evidence of clear comprehension of the underlying principles of all methodology used. I wish to see evidence of validation and quality control for all methodologies where these can be appropriately derived. I expect to see an adequate and reasoned statement of any statistical methodology used. It is not sufficient simply to list methods; I must understand why you have used those particular methods for your data. I expect to see, either at the end of the methods section or in a formal statement at the very start of the work, an unambiguous statement of how much of the practical work was actually done by you personally. Very few theses these days are produced from work done only by a single investigator without the active collaboration of one or several others. Teamwork is as important in medicine as it is in science and must be acknowledged.

Results

In considering the results section of a thesis, I look for information about pilot studies and how the data from these have been incorporated into the main study. The results section must be written in English and not 'computerese' and must be comprehensive but succinct. Again, the ability to summarise is extremely important. It is unusual for all hypotheses tested to be supported and I normally expect to see some 'negative' as well as 'positive' results. Provided that the work has been logically designed to test a clearly stated hypothesis and has thereafter been done in a proper manner, a statement that the null hypothesis was supported has just as much importance as one that it was rejected. I do not expect to see interpretations of data in the results section of a thesis.

While you may wish to report work done in collaboration with others in the main body of your thesis, I do not expect to see data derived by somebody else presented in the results section. If it is necessary for the interpretation of your data, then it should be given in the discussion and clearly identified as having been performed by a collaborator.

Non-text material

I look for clear and well presented figures, tables and other non-text material. These can help the reader enormously and it is well worth spending the time to learn how to present your data professionally. I do not, however, like to see data presented in more than one format. Thus, I wish to see data either in the text or in a table or in a figure; you should decide which is the most effective form of presentation. I expect a careful approach to references in the text to figures and tables. Figures and tables themselves should be accompanied by informative legends but, again, these should not recapitulate the text.

Discussion

The discussion is among the most important parts of the thesis. It is here that I look for evidence of the candidate's intellectual ability. The acquisition of data for a thesis could in many cases be done every bit as well (and sometimes considerably better) by a competent fully trained technician. What should distinguish the doctoral student is that they have devised the work, carried it through and interpreted it in the light of their own background knowledge.

I do not expect to see a recapitulation of the results in the discussion section. This is tedious for me and wastes trees. The discussion is where I look for your statement of how you think your work relates to the work of others:

- How does it extend, expand, amplify such work?
- Can you convince me that it is novel and a genuine addition to the corpus of knowledge?
- Are you honest in your discussion of difficulties and discrepancies?

I look for evidence of self-criticism as well as criticism of the work of others. I expect to see a formal consideration of potential sources of error, both initially realised and those which came to light subsequently. I then expect to see how you attempted to minimise those of which you were aware initially and how you would redesign the work were you to be repeating it, in the light of problems which arose during the work. I hope to see a statement or statements about specific areas suitable for future work. A bland statement that 'more research is evidently required' merely annoys me. If you are not excited by the implications of your work, it is improbable that others will be.

References

The reference list should contain all references mentioned in the text and not contain any references not mentioned in the text. Examiners vary as to what proportion of references they will initially check. However, as soon as I become aware of a missing reference, my index of suspicion rises and I proceed to check a higher proportion. It is sloppy for a candidate not to have got their referencing right and immediately makes me wonder whether they have been sloppy in other aspects of the work. The format of the references should conform to that of other theses within your university. I expect the candidate to read every reference to which they refer and if I have any suspicions about this, I will test it at the *viva* (see below). I also expect candidates to have read the full papers and not merely the abstracts as displayed on

Medline. These can sometimes be inaccurate and positively misleading and, again, it is a sloppy habit. I look for evidence of reading of the original research articles with only minimal use of reviews.

Acknowledgements

I like to see generosity in acknowledgements. Many people will have helped you, both directly and indirectly in your thesis work and you should be prepared to acknowledge this.

Presentation

The presentation of your thesis is something else which I will take into account as a small but important matter. Sloppy presentation suggests to me the possibility that the work itself will also have been sloppily done. For example, poor grammar and semiliterate spelling both annoy me *per se* and make me suspicious about standards in other areas. Examiners list typographical and spelling errors and demand revision of these as well as other matters. If you do not take a pride in your thesis, nobody else is likely to.

The *viva voce* examination

Once an examiner has read a thesis, they are usually asked to write their own report on the thesis. These will be collated by the internal examiner who then has the responsibility of organising the *viva voce* examination. Not all universities require a *viva* for all research degrees. However, they are very common and will always be held if the examiners have to decide between the options of rejection or re-writing after reading the thesis. The candidate should be able to display a wide general knowledge of the field of the study in which their thesis lies. I view with considerable disfavour the candidate who says brightly 'Well, it took me five years to write up and I haven't had time to keep up with the field' when displaying abysmal ignorance of the current literature. The work is being submitted for a higher degree and your own standards should be commensurate with this. You should expect to defend your work at the *viva* but not to try to cover up weakness. I view the *viva* as being important and will spend as long as I think necessary over it. However, if I am the internal examiner, I will usually keep relatively quiet during the *viva* since this is usually regarded as being primarily a matter for the external examiner(s). It is most unusual, but not unheard of, for the adviser/supervisor to be present in the same room as that in which the *viva* is being held. However, it is usual that they are available within the department or on the end of a telephone to clarify any ambiguities which the examiners may wish to raise after the *viva*.

Outcome

After the *viva*, the examiners then come to a conclusion about the outcome. At the worst, is outright rejection if the work is fundamentally unsound, trivial and/or unsalvageable. Fortunately, such a decision is rare. In my experience, the examiners will be in complete accord about this outcome. When this happens, it is usual for the internal examiner subsequently to have a meeting with the head of department and adviser/supervisor to try to determine how the work could have been allowed to get to the stage of submission without its inadequacies being identified and remedied.

A weak PhD (or DPhil) submission may be rejected for the higher degree but revision recommended which will make it suitable for the award of MPhil. The PhD is usually accomplished in three to four years and, in other than exceptional circumstances, one would expect that at least MPhil level should be attainable. The MD (or DM) by research is usually undertaken in a period of two years and there is at present no 'fall-back' degree if an inadequate standard has been reached.

If the work is basically of an acceptable quality but contains weaknesses of analysis and/or interpretation or requires (a small amount of) additional experimental or observational work, the candidate will be offered the option of remedial work with resubmission within a set period. Such an offer should be taken up as it implies that, provided that the work is undertaken to a satisfactory standard, the degree will be awarded. When this option is offered, it is important to remain within the time deadlines given. The examiners are experienced people who will not be asking the unreasonable or impossible, but are also aware that the longer such revision is allowed to drag on, the less likely it is that final resubmission will be made.

The thesis work can be accepted if the work and *viva* outcome are satisfactory, usually with a requirement that typographical and other minor errors be corrected before final approval. Such final approval is usually given by the internal examiner without further reference to the external examiner(s).

In some universities, the possibility of the higher degree being awarded with a distinction exists. I would only recommend such an award in truly exceptional circumstances where I was convinced of the candidate's own originality of thought and excellence of work. I would never countenance such an award without a *viva*.

When the examiners have arrived at their decision of the outcome of the examination, they prepare a report for the head of department and faculty board, in addition to the individual reports which they have prepared on the thesis itself. Where more than minor revision is required, the internal examiner is usually responsible for passing on the examiners' requirements to the candidate.

I know that this all sounds very formal and legalistic. However, the process is an attempt to maintain the standard of the 'currency' of higher level academic research in the United Kingdom. It helps no one to allow substandard work through the system. At the time when you submit your thesis, you should know more about your topic than anyone else in the world and should be excited by it. It is up to you to convince the examiners of the value of the work.

Index